CW00384800

A PATENTED
HEART DISEASE
CURE
THAT WORKS

A PATENTED
HEART DISEASE
CURE
THAT WORKS

SECOND EDITION

**WHAT YOUR DOCTOR MAY NOT KNOW.
WHAT BIG PHARMA HOPES YOU DON'T FIND OUT!**

DAVID H. LEAKE

© 2012, 2018 David H. Leake

Second Edition
Revised and Corrected

All rights reserved. No part of this book may be reproduced or transmitted in any form or by any means, electronic or mechanical, including photocopying, recording, or by any information storage and retrieval system, except in the case of brief quotations embodied in critical articles and reviews, without prior written permission of the publisher.

Disclaimer

None of what is provided here is intended to diagnose or treat any ailment. I am not a physician, nor should anything I write be taken as medical advice. I am simply reporting my own experience -- plus that which I have learned from books and several Internet sites (referenced throughout and in Appendix C). While I believe wholeheartedly in the curative powers of the ideas presented here, everything I have written is strictly a layman's opinion. Nothing here should be considered a substitute for the advice of your doctor. Rather, you should use it as a point of discussion with him or her.

I hope you find a heart doctor who is as open to this discussion as three of mine have been. While they remained skeptical, they have been willing to monitor my condition and make recommendations. My doctor in Winter Park, FL, was willing, for instance, to let me experiment with eliminating Lipitor (thank goodness) and stop taking two blood pressure medications -- both of which proved unnecessary. My current doctor in Bradenton, FL, is more skeptical, but we have reached an accord – no statins or other drugs in exchange for my taking a baby aspirin every third day, at least for now.

ISBN Paperback: 978-1-7324064-0-7
ISBN eBook: 978-1-7324064-1-4

Interior Design: Ghislain Viau – Creative Publishing Book Design

This book is dedicated to the memory my deceased parents, Howard and Beulah Leake, my grandfather, Daniel Leake, and all the millions of other victims of coronary artery disease. Until my generation, none had a chance to beat this killer. Now, we do.

Special thanks to those who contributed their time and effort to helping me compile and edit this, my first book, and to all the experts who graciously permitted me to quote them.

IN MEMORIUM

Duane Graveline, MD, MPH, former USAF Flight Surgeon, Former NASA Astronaut/Medical Researcher, Retired Family Doctor, passed away on September 5, 2016, at the age of 85. You can read details of his life at *http://tinyurl.com/yaptmq96*.

He believed to the end his declining health and ultimate demise were due to statin drugs (Reference: *http://tinyurl.com/y8294xrd*). "Space Doc" was a mentor to me and many others who believe statins cause irreversible damage to our ability to remember, and to our overall health. He fought Big Pharma with his writings, his website (*www.SpaceDoc. com*) and his books. His medical research for NASA, along with some of the devices he developed, are still aiding astronauts to this day.

Doctor Graveline's website is a veritable Who's Who of medical professionals and researchers who have come to distrust all the hype about statin drugs and their supposed benefits. Much of what I have learned on this topic has come from the work of this group of mavericks. I encourage you to explore SpaceDoc's website as well as his links to work by the others displayed on his home page. A treasure trove of his and their reference materials can be found here: *http://www.spacedoc. com/sitemap.php*, and on the website of The International Network of Cholesterol Skeptics (THINCS), at *https://www.thincs.org/*.

For instance, Dr. Graveline's extensive report, "Statins and CoQ10 Deficiency," can be found at *http://tinyurl.com/y84s66rg*.

A note about the format: This is a "cross-over" book, if you will. It falls between print books and "eBooks." There is substantial information within its pages to convey the main points. However, due to the richness of content to be found these days on the Internet, it seemed only appropriate to include live links to extended resources for those reading this in digital form. This book is also available in digital format, where it includes those live links. You can also view those live links by visiting my website, *www.AWorldWithoutHeartDisease.com*. I don't want to hear another word about "old people" (like me) being unable to cope in this digital age, because the majority of us certainly can.

References in this book to websites often take the form of "http:// tinyurl.com/," followed by a series of letters and numbers. You can type them as a URL, or click as a link in digital versions of the book. This format is used as a way to truncate excessively long web addresses. To learn more, visit *http://tinyurl.com/.*

First Printing: April 2012
Revised Update: 2018

Special Note: Because this book was first created for e-readers in electronic book format, you will find Internet link references scattered throughout. I decided to leave them in the print version for those who would still like the option of looking up further information on the Internet. They can also be accessed as live links in the "Resources" section of my website, http://aworldwithoutheartdisease.com/resources.

Throughout the book I have employed "TinyURL" versions of website links to save space. For posterity, I have added complete URLs in Appendix C.

TABLE OF CONTENTS

ABOUT THOSE TWO PHOTOS OF MY OWN HEART'S ARTERIES REPEATED THROUGHOUT THIS BOOK:

Both images are X-rays of my heart's arteries, taken during an exploratory angiogram conducted at Florida Hospital Orlando on July 27, 2011. Unfortunately, I have no "before" images. I turned 70 years old in January 2012. Nurses in the "cath lab" said they hoped their own arteries right then looked as good as mine. The interventional cardiology specialist who performed the procedure proclaimed my heart healthy (*"free of obstructive disease,"* were his written words) as did my family doctor, based on the cardiologist's report.

The upper photo is of my Left Anterior Descending (LAD) artery bundle, commonly known to heart doctors as "the widow maker." At one point, it contained a blockage of 85 percent. Later, my heart became home to three metal mesh stents. The only damage this cardiologist could now find involved those stents.

The lower photo displays the clean arteries on the back side of my heart. That straight line is actually the X-ray image of the catheter that was inserted through my thigh, into my femoral artery and then threaded into my heart. Through it, contrasting dye was injected that would then light up the X-rays. Dark spots are intersections, where a branch attaches to the main vessel. They are dark because we are looking into the trunk of a wide open vessel, so the camera picks up a greater amount of dye in the blood passing through that point.

My change in heart health occurred *after* 17 years of bad reactions to every statin drug (Lipitor was the last and the worst). It was only after I had run out of statin options that I turned in desperation to searching the Internet. That's how I discovered the 1994 patent that changed my life. It might change yours, and that's what this book is about.

INTRODUCTION

"Treating the symptoms of nutritional deficiency with drugs becomes nothing more than an experiment, where we get to observe the toxic effects on a malnourished body."
—Author Unknown

"The current way doctors treat heart disease is misguided because they treat the risk factors not the causes. To think we can treat heart disease by lowering cholesterol, lowering blood pressure and lowering blood sugar with medication is like mopping up the floor while the sink overflows."
—Mark Hyman, MD, in the Huffington Post
(https://tinyurl.com/yce3be5c) Updated May 04, 2017

My father's father died in 1941, a year before I was born. A doctor said he had "fat around the heart," and he needed to exercise. So he went for a jog, came home, and dropped dead at age 56 of a massive coronary. I have lived with that story all my life. In fact, every male in my father's family going back at least three generations has died from heart disease. My mother did, too.

I was just 48 in 1990, when I received what I assumed to be my own death sentence. Tests revealed an 85 percent blockage in the LAD, my heart's Left Anterior Descending artery, the one doctors call "the widow maker." A doctor opened the artery in a procedure called angioplasty, by pressing the built-up plaque against the artery wall. But I spent the next twenty years of my life being cautious about exercise, and fearing "the big one."

By 2003 my heart disease had spread. In another angioplasty procedure, I was given three stents, metal mesh cylinders, to prop parts of my arteries open. And, on January 9, 2004, my then-heart doctor issued me a letter of "permanent limitation" of activities. He stated, "This patient has severe multivessel coronary disease and has undergone multivessel coronary angioplasty" (see page xvii).

Yet, in a "final report" on results of an angiogram conducted July 27, 2011, an expert cardiologist reported my heart to be "*free of obstructive disease.*" In fact, he concluded, the only remaining damaged areas in my heart involved those three stents placed there in 2003. A nurse standing next to him said she hoped her own arteries were as clean as mine. Reason for the procedure that day? Florida heat … not a heart attack.

I had run out of hope around 2007, after Lipitor, the last statin drug available to me at that time, ended up causing severe side effects, just like all the others I'd tried since 1989. I felt all I could do at that point was let my heart disease run its course until it killed me.

So, imagine my surprise when an extensive Internet search led me to U.S. Patent #5278189 – filed in 1994 by American scientist Linus Pauling and German medical doctor Matthias Rath. It claimed to be *a cure for heart disease* (technically titled "Prevention and treatment of occlusive cardiovascular disease with ascorbate and substances that inhibit the binding of lipoprotein (A)").

It's a patent Big Pharma, the American Medical Association and American Heart Association have known about *since 1994.* None of them has shown the least bit of interest. In fact, they have sought to diminish it and to denigrate its authors, one of them a two-time Nobel Prize winning scientist who had nothing to gain by its publication. There's no money in it. At least, there's no big money. This is a cheap cure based on over the counter supplements. The two inventors placed it in the public domain, and no public or private agency has even seen fit to give it an adequate clinical trial.

After three years on this regimen, my documented "severe multivessel coronary disease" was GONE – as in "*free of obstructive disease*," the interventional cardiologist's words in July 2011 – and I am angry. Why have I and millions of others suffered needlessly for decades, when a cure was available? Why have so many of your relatives and mine died from an epidemic that could have been prevented? Why have so many suffered side effects of statin drugs? And, why will I have to live the rest of my life with damage caused by stents my heart never would have needed had this inexpensive cure for heart disease been widely supported? (More on the long term dangers of stents, from my recent personal experience, in the new Chapter Two of this 2018 edition)

As you read this book you will learn:

- Coronary Artery Disease can be reversed, cured and prevented
- cholesterol level is unrelated to heart disease
- statin drugs do not reduce death rates due to heart disease
- side effects of statin drugs are far more common than is being reported, and include permanent muscle damage, brain damage, loss of memory, kidney damage and more.

Imagine the lives that can be extended, the suffering that can be prevented, when more people learn there already exists a safe and inexpensive cure for heart disease.

This book is for them, and YOU.

January 9, 2004
Re: David H Leake
Date of Birth: 01/29/1942
OHC Chart #: 039138

To Whom It May Concern:

This patient has severe multivessel coronary disease and has undergone multivessel coronary angioplasty. When over stressed he developed angina because of disease that cannot be treated. At this time I feel he should work no more than 40 hours a week with a maximum of 8 hours a day. Pushing beyond this is too stressful for his medical condition. Please do not hesitate to contact me if I can be of further assistance. This is a permanent limitation beginning at the time of his angioplasty in August 2003.

Sincerely,

George E. Andreae, M.D., F.A.C.C.
GEA/mh

Copied from the original letter written by my then-cardiologist and re-sized due to format restrictions.

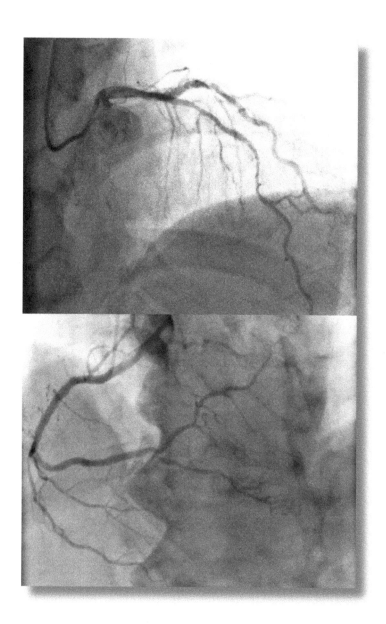

CHAPTER ONE

THE END

Everyone likes to skip to the end of a book to see how it turns out. In this book, the end is so important I am placing it at the beginning.

When people learn I reversed my own heart disease they want me to cut to the chase. "How'd you do it?" they want to know, hoping they or a loved one can do the same. So, while I hope you will read the remainder – to learn just how this works, and a lot more – here is the secret formula.

1. Massive doses of Vitamin C *(as Ascorbic Acid)*, **6,000mg to 18,000mg daily in divided doses.** *Take with or before meals, i.e., 2 to 3 times daily.* At least for the first few weeks, take as much as you can, and never mind the FDA "daily values"; their silly 60 milligrams is enough to suppress the external symptoms of scurvy, nothing more. Linus Pauling, who patented this cure, along with German medical doctor

Matthias Rath, was reportedly taking 18,000 milligrams (18 grams) per day to prove the safety of Vitamin C. He died at the ripe old age of 93 (of prostate cancer, not heart disease), just a few months after obtaining his patent. Pauling's prescription for you, in phase 1: "Vitamin C to bowel tolerance," taken at 3 to 4 hour intervals.

That tolerance level was one I did not want to tolerate, personally. However, I was able to take 10,000 milligrams (10 grams), which I did for the first couple months. My maintenance level had been 6 to 9 grams divided in three doses, morning, noon and night.

2018 update. Late last year, at age 75, I bit my tongue severely and was prescribed a liquid diet for at least one week. I cut back on most of my supplements as well, keeping only those for heart and memory. This seemed like a good time to experiment with vitamin C tolerance, so I began increasing my C levels in increments. At 12 grams per day something surprising happened. My hemorrhoids stopped bleeding. After a few weeks at 15 grams, another surprise. The skin on my hands – which typically gets thinner with age – appears slightly thicker. Enough, at least, that as of this writing those veins which had stood out as bluish lines are once again flesh color. All of this suggests increased intake of vitamin C is benefitting my entire body, not just my heart.

Fifteen grams, at first, seemed to be my personal optimal level; my constipation had lessened without engendering C's one known side effect with high doses, diarrhea. After a few weeks at 15 grams, though, "bowel tolerance" and Montezuma caught up with me. As I write this, I am again tinkering to find my own tolerable level of high dose C.

After my failed adventure at 15 grams of ascorbic acid crystals, I've returned to 500 milligram tablets. While taking the crystals, though, my preferred option to reduce stomach irritation was to mix a ratio of two parts ascorbic acid powder with one part baking soda in a tall glass of water. Another option would be sodium ascorbate because it has a neutral pH; however, in the large quantities discussed here, its sodium content might play havoc with blood pressure.

Vitamin C is absolutely the foundation for this heart cure. Taking anything less than 6,000 milligrams per day is cheating yourself – and your heart. You can buy it on line or at most local grocery stores or pharmacies. If you have difficulty swallowing the big 1,000 milligram tablets, try doubling up on the smaller 500 milligram ones. That works for me.

NOTE: If "bowel tolerance" becomes an issue with vitamin C at levels lower than those desired, other options are available that might help. Non-acidic Ester C (calcium ascorbate) tablets are available in stores and on line. Liposomal vitamin C is said to be absorbed better; I have told some of its makers, though, that its cost is prohibitive for most people at the volumes discussed here. It, too, is available on line, or there are even instructions you can find on the Internet for the tedious – if less costly – process of making Liposomal vitamin C in your own kitchen. I'm dubious the average person has either the skill or the time involved to do that.

2. L-Lysine 3,000mg to 6,000mg daily in divided doses. I take it at the same time as my Vitamin C. L-Lysine is an essential amino acid that helps remove plaque from the walls of heart arteries.

3. L-Proline 3,000mg to 6,000mg daily in divided doses. This was later recommended by Pauling, Rath and others to work in conjunction with Vitamin C and Lysine. If you are unable to find L-Proline locally, it has been available on line and at health stores such as GNC.

The vitamin C strengthens heart arteries (more on that later). Lysine and Proline molecules bond with built up plaque and gradually flush it from your system.

So, there you have the bare basics.

THE END
(Just kidding)

2018 Cautionary Note. In late summer and fall of 2014, I developed a condition my then-gastroenterologist claimed was esophagitis. That doctor – who refused to believe a word of this book – claimed the cause was my massive intake of vitamin C; she claimed the acid (vitamin C, after all, is ascorbic acid) was destroying my throat (my daughter-in-law, an RN, said another cause might have been my decade long habit of swallowing 30+ supplements at a single gulp); this doctor insisted I stop all vitamin C and begin taking a proton pump inhibitor (PPI). One possible side effect of PPIs is "microscopic colitis," which I developed in spades, along with its related bouts of diarrhea. Another PPI side effect can be *heart disease*. Go figure.

As you will learn in Chapter 2, I stopped the vitamin C at my peril and nearly died – only to be told later, by a more knowledgeable gastroenterologist that vitamin C is too weak an acid to have caused my throat problems in the first place.

Reference: "Vitamin C Material: Where to Start, What to Watch" – Commentary by Tom Taylor (https://tinyurl.com/ybrrh8gt). Rightfully slams – in my opinion – those who have taken over the Linus Pauling Institute at Oregon State University since Pauling's death; they appear to have been cowed by Big Pharma.

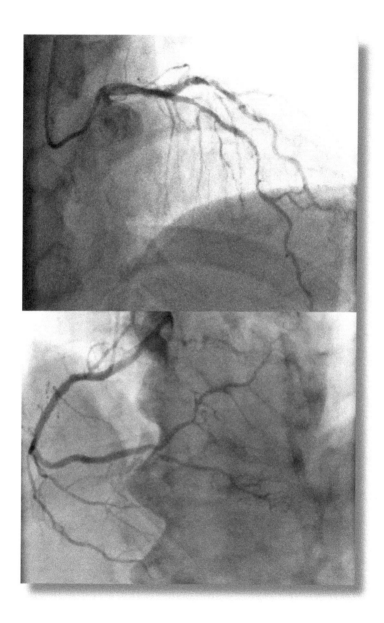

CHAPTER TWO

WHAT HAPPENS IF
I STOP THIS PROTOCOL?

Early in 2014 a visitor to my website, AWorldWithoutHeartDisease.com, asked, "When can I stop the Pauling/Rath protocol?"

I was unable to answer from any personal experience, but I repeated Linus Pauling's admonition, "Never miss a day."

Well, now I know – from personal experience – and the answer isn't pretty. In short, Pauling was correct. This is a story of stupidity on my part, with real life consequences

In December 2015, after a couple days' vigorous walking at Orlando theme parks, I ended up with two new stents in my left anterior descending artery – "LAD" for short. It's the artery doctors call "the widow maker." Those stents were placed inside an existing pair from 2003 that were said to be failing. And I was prescribed blood thinners, just as with my previous stent procedures. This had nothing to do with the Pauling/Rath protocol, as you will see in a minute. Bear with me.

Looking back, from December of 2013 to the summer of 2014, I was having trouble with a near-continuous dry cough that could only be controlled with a prescription drug called Tessalon Pearls. Our family doctor suggested I see a gastroenterologist.

My first encounter with this GI doc on August 4, 2014, should have been a warning. As I always do when seeing a new MD, I gave this doctor (whom we'll call Dr. A) a copy of this book. Doctor A almost went ballistic, denying my "supposed" cure, and giving no credence to the Pauling/Rath protocol. "It must have been a change in diet or something," was said dismissively. Whereupon I should have ended the conversation and walked out. Sadly, I did not.

Dr. A conducted an upper GI endoscopy to check out my esophagus. The initial conclusion was that I had GERD, Gastroesophageal Reflux Disease, brought on by "too much stomach acid." The likely cause of that was – wait for it – *excess amounts of vitamin C.* I was strongly advised to cease taking C altogether, and given a prescription for Prevacid, a proton pump inhibitor.

Later, in a follow-up visit for my wife, I chimed in about my own case and mentioned the finding of GERD. "You don't have GERD," Dr. A retorted. "You have esophagitis." I looked it up and found it can lead to Barrett's Esophagus and, ultimately, cancer in a minority of cases.

Elsewhere in this book, I point out that every member of my family – except one – going back a couple generations died from coronary artery disease. Wouldn't you know? That one, Dad's mother, died from cancer of the esophagus.

So, while my focus had for decades been on heart disease, it was suddenly shifted like a laser to this other risk. Needless to say, I followed this doctor's advice, and gave up the Pauling/Rath protocol even though Pauling had warned, "Never miss a day."

Meanwhile, in reading up on Prevacid and all other proton pump inhibitors (PPIs), I kept coming across FDA advisories *to not use these drugs more than 14 days* **in any given year**. When I broached this to my gastroenterologist, Dr. A brusquely replied, "That's only if you are not under a doctor's supervision. *You are under a doctor's supervision now.*" And then I did not see this doctor for many months.

When I did see Dr. A again, I was complaining about chronic diarrhea. I was scheduled for a colonoscopy that determined I was suffering from something called "microscopic colitis." Guess what? A search of the Internet for side effects of proton pump inhibitors reveals microscopic colitis can be one of them. So maybe the FDA knew something.

At this point, my allergist – when I mentioned all this to him – suggested I try switching myself to over-the-counter Pepcid. He subtly implied I might want to get a second opinion from another gastroenterologist.

And that is what I did … way too late, and about six weeks after the 2015 installation of my new heart stents inside two existing ones that had plugged up.

Meanwhile, a side "benefit," if you will, of my experience was a resulting image from the angiogram taken during the installation of my two new heart stents inside existing ones.

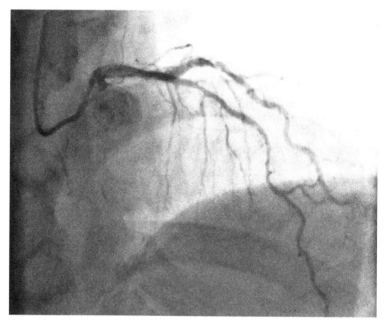

Notice the similarity, for the most part, between this image and those shown throughout this book taken in 2011. In other words, the Pauling/Rath Vitamin C protocol was still working four years later. It remains possible that the buildup inside two of my three original 2003 stents was scar overgrowth caused by the existence of those two stents.

As one of my previous heart doctors said, "If it weren't for those stents, I would have you on no heart medications at all."

My new gastroenterologist (Dr. B) received all records about my esophagus from Dr. A. These included images from the endoscopy of my throat, clinical notes, plus lab results from biopsies.

Dr. B's words struck like thunder: "You don't have esophagitis. You never had it. You have some throat irritation. It may be from reflux, or post nasal drip, or a combination. But I see no reason you should not restart vitamin C."

Vitamin C, Dr. B pointed out, *is too weak an acid to significantly increase stomach acid levels*. After all, the acid in your stomach is hydrochloric, one of the strongest known to man.

And the *diarrhea*? When I saw a family doctor, complaining of a pain in my side, she had me fast for a day in preparation for a CT scan. I felt better at the end of that day, and decided on my own to continue my fast for a second day.

Fasting did the trick. The *pain subsided. Better yet, **the diarrhea stopped.** And the scan came back negative, suggesting I'd had some sort of temporary blockage in my intestines.*

Needless to say, I resumed the Pauling/Rath protocol, returning to a daily regimen of eight or nine grams of Vitamin C in four divided doses daily; plus one gram of L-Lysine three times daily, and 500 mg of L-Proline morning and night. As I write this, in the spring of 2018 (now age 76), my current heart doctor has blackmailed me into continuing baby aspirin as a blood thinner. It's either that, he said, or find a new heart doctor. We did reach a negotiated settlement, of sorts: I argued him down to one baby aspirin every third day (since even he acknowledges it lingers in your blood stream that long), and no other blood thinners, period. Even so, I was still dealing with those annoying side effects of skin bruises on both arms.

I fully believe all this did not have to happen. Oh, if I had only listened to Linus Pauling, and never missed a day.

Note 1: at my recent increase to 15 grams of C each day, the bruising mostly disappeared. As described in Chapter 1, though, that dosage took me beyond my personal tolerance level.

Note 2: A follower on my YouTube page suggested there might have been another cause of my stent blockages ... one beyond the control of Vitamin C. "Drug eluting" metal stents – the kind I and millions of others have – can cause scar tissue to build up inside them. However, the longest time from implantation for a blockage to occur is thought to be about six years; mine were in place twice that long, so my likely culprit remains restenosis, or gradual build-up of plaque inside the existing stents.

My YouTube follower's concern is not an issue to view lightly, however. Because heart arteries are forever expanding, contracting and moving – and because a rigid stent can restrict that movement and cause inflammation – that can lead, in some patients, to tissue from the artery growing into and inside of drug eluting stents. That is why, for many heart patients (present party included), stents may mean a lifelong blood thinning medication.

This has been a sufficient enough problem that, in 2016, the FDA approved a new self-dissolving heart stent from Abbott Laboratories. The new stent remains intact for one year. Then, over the next two years, it dissolves and is absorbed by the body. Already sold in Europe and Asia, Abbott's Absorb stent holds the hope that risks of future complications from stents will be reduced. Long term safety of the new stents won't be known until enough have been implanted to see the results, probably in 2022.

Note 3: The condition I was led to believe started all this – supposedly, "too much stomach acid," leading to throat irritation and a persistent cough – may have been just the reverse. A book I recently discovered – Why Stomach Acid Is Good for You (Amazon Kindle, http://tinyurl.com/y73jyudm) by Jonathan V. Wright M.D., and Lane Lenard Ph.D. – suggests senior citizens (like me) most often suffer from too little stomach acid.

Sadly, I will never be able to report to you whether Wright and Lenard are correct. First off, they caution never to begin their protocol – which involves ingesting capsules of hydrochloric acid – if you are taking aspirin or other blood thinners. Secondly, although my current gastroenterologist has invested in the equipment to test acid levels in patients' stomachs, it sits unused in his closet. Reason? At this time, no health insurance company will cover the testing procedure, which is quite costly.

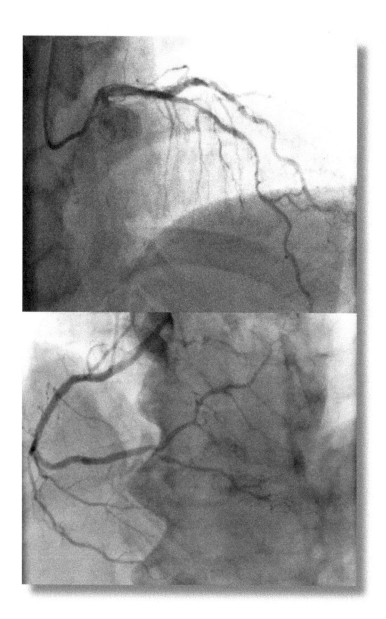

CHAPTER THREE

WAS LINUS PAULING NUTS?

To my everlasting shame, I was not impressed with Linus Pauling when I met him. He was an old coot (63 at the time, multiple years younger than I am now) and had only thirty productive years left ahead of him. Interesting, isn't it, how our perspectives change?

Pauling had an odd Oregon accent (i.e., distinctly NOT like mine from New England), and he wore that little poufy French beret. I was only 22, had just graduated from Boston University, and didn't know what I didn't know.

Our paths crossed in 1964, on the campus of Bowdoin College in Brunswick, Maine. I had been lucky enough to land my first job, as assistant director of news services, at Bowdoin. It was, and still is, one of the most prestigious small liberal arts colleges in the country.

That summer, the college opened its new dormitory for seniors, a mini-high rise tower dubbed, simply, "The Senior

Center" back then. It was more than a dorm, though. It also housed suites for visiting lecturers – distinguished guests who would stay several weeks, and open their doors in the evenings for impromptu gatherings of students, faculty and staff.

Linus Pauling was one of the very first guest lecturers when classes began that fall. I was introduced to him at a party honoring his arrival, and we would pass occasionally on the campus pathways. He always sported that beret, and was usually walking with an entourage of Bowdoin's brightest science majors hanging on his every word.

I heard him speak once. Gibberish, it seemed to me, because he was speaking in the language of brilliant scholars. My all-time favorite cartoon from the *New Yorker* magazine sums it up best; it depicted a scholarly gent looking at a blue collar Joe, and the caption read, "I'd love to explain it to you in Layman's Language, *but I don't know any Layman's Language*."

That was the gulf between me and Linus Pauling. It was my shortcoming, not his.

At the time of his death in 1994, Pauling held as many as 48 honorary Ph.D.s. Wikipedia (https://en.wikipedia.org/wiki/Linus_Pauling) reports, "Pauling is one of only four individuals to have won more than one Nobel Prize. He is one of only two people awarded Nobel Prizes in different fields (the Chemistry and Peace prizes), the other being Marie Curie (the Chemistry and Physics prizes), and the only person awarded two unshared (Nobel) prizes."

Quoting, again, from Wikipedia, "Pauling was included in a list of the 20 greatest scientists of all time by the magazine New Scientist, with Albert Einstein being the only other scientist from the twentieth century on the list. Gautam R. Desiraju, the author of the Millennium Essay in Nature, claimed that Pauling was one of the greatest thinkers and visionaries of the millennium, along with Galileo, Newton, and Einstein. Pauling is notable for the diversity of his interests: quantum mechanics, inorganic chemistry, organic chemistry, protein structure, molecular biology, and medicine. In all these fields, and especially on the boundaries between them, he made decisive contributions. His work on chemical bonding marks the beginning of modern quantum chemistry, and many of his contributions like hybridization and electronegativity have become part of standard chemistry textbooks."

No wonder I couldn't understand him.

However, in the mid-1970's, when I was suffering from back-to-back colds, I turned to a new book for help. It was Pauling's *Vitamin C and the Common Cold*, later re-issued as *Vitamin C, the Common Cold and the Flu*. I remembered the man I had met a dozen years earlier. By then I was more aware of his fame and his intellect. I expected his book would help me, and did it ever!

I began taking Vitamin C as Pauling recommended, and my colds went away. I'd had seldom as much as a sniffle since. Little wonder, then, that my mind was open to his ideas when I came across his name again in 2007.

It was in the 1970's, also, that Pauling began investigating with several medical doctors the effects of vitamin C in extending the lives of terminal cancer patients – those hopeless souls whose diseases had been declared "untreatable." Their findings indicated terminal patients on chemotherapy alone died in about six months, while those terminal cancer patients who took only very high doses of intravenous Vitamin C remained alive *1 to 12 years* longer. Their studies were replicated in Scotland, Canada and Japan. Cancer treatment medications have improved since then, so their effectiveness might be better than vitamin C in most cases today. Still, there are cancer patients hoping to gain time by taking massive doses of C.*

All this talk about the benefits of Vitamin C was of concern to the pharmaceutical industry (more on this in Chapter 8). Perhaps it was because profits to be made producing natural Vitamin C are woefully less than those to be had from patentable synthetic drugs. It was at that point they began a campaign to discredit Pauling and other advocates for this vitamin.

It seems odd Pauling's competence could be challenged beginning in the 1970's, yet as late as 1990 he was still giving recorded interviews (some available on YouTube) about his ongoing studies of the atomic nucleus.

View one of the last known videos of him at age 91, and decide for yourself: https://tinyurl.com/yb2dpjbm. In this video he speaks about vitamin C – uninterrupted and without notes – for more than an hour, not even stopping for a sip of water.

More information on efforts to discredit Pauling can be seen at https://tinyurl.com/ydzykbua

Pauling was born February 28, 1901, in Portland, Oregon. He died of prostate cancer on August 19, 1994, in Big Sur, CA. He is buried in Oswego Pioneer Cemetery, Lake Oswego, OR, near where he lived as a child. Thanks to him and the American M.D., Thomas Levy, New Zealand became the first country in the world to recognize vitamin C as a legitimate medical treatment. Someone there produced a tribute video to Pauling that can be seen here: https://tinyurl.com/nahbrtl.

To answer my own question, No, I do not think Linus Pauling was nuts.

§

*(Note: Vitamin C's potential for treating some forms of cancer is on the front burner again – at least in non-pharmaceutical circles. A team of British researchers documented that taking massive oral doses of vitamin C can, indeed, increase its concentrations in your blood stream, far beyond the ~280 μm L^{-1} previously thought to be the maximum possible. Writing in the Journal of Nutritional and Environmental Medicine in 2008 they reported ". . . a short *in vitro* treatment of human Burkitt's lymphoma cells with ascorbate, at 400 μm L^{-1}, has been shown to result in ~50% cancer cell death. Using frequent oral doses, an equivalent plasma level could be sustained indefinitely. Thus, oral vitamin C has potential for use as a non-toxic, sustainable, therapeutic agent." Read more at https://tinyurl.com/ycmfs4e8.)

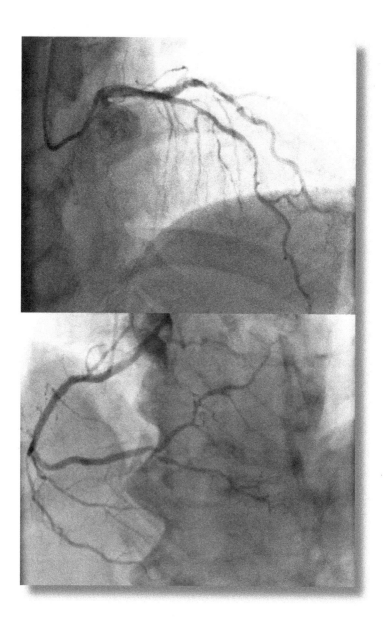

CHAPTER FOUR

WHAT DID PAULING AND RATH LEARN ABOUT HEART DISEASE?

What if everything you thought you knew about heart disease was *wrong*? What if cholesterol was not "good" or "bad?" What if LDL was a life saving friend, not "the enemy?" What if something else accounted for atherosclerotic blockages, i.e. "heart disease?" And, what if you didn't need any toxic drugs to stop or even reverse heart disease, and maybe even prevent strokes?

In the early 1900's, medicine was at a crossroads. Natural healers, "naturopaths," believed in warding off disease by strengthening the body through the use of herbs and minerals, among other things. A lot of what they practiced – blood letting, poultices, and reliance on various natural ingredients – could only be explained as tradition. It was a form of medicine passed down through generations.

Medical doctors (M.D.'s) and laboratory scientists, meanwhile, were moving towards the use of patentable synthetic chemicals to treat disease. With the advent of penicillin and other "miracle drugs" during WWII the big money went into pharmaceuticals. And by the 1950's, the American Medical Association and "Big Pharma" were waging campaigns to wipe out naturopathic "heretics." By the late 50's, naturopathy was licensed in only five states.

That was the way things stood until the 1970's, when a third front in human health care opened. Call it a new approach or perhaps naturopathy on steroids. Pauling coined a term for it: Orthomolecular Nutrition (https://tinyurl.com/ya7pw89c). At any rate, a champion came along, one supporting an alternative to reliance only on pharmaceuticals to cure some of our ills. This was no lightweight 1900's "remedy" pusher. It was double Nobel Prize winner (1954 and 1962) Linus Pauling. He was among the first to work in the fields of quantum chemistry (http://tinyurl.com/yaz2btg9) and molecular biology (http://tinyurl.com/lhclspj). He was a scientist with impeccable credentials. He took us into the inner workings of the trillions of individual cells that make up our bodies. He was able to explain – in scientific terms, not old-time hocus pocus – how keeping all of those individual cells healthy could strengthen every organ and keep our whole bodies healthy. And, he explored an alternative path to treating some of our most serious diseases.

As Linus Pauling explains in his 1986 book, *How to Live Longer and Feel Better (*https://tinyurl.com/ya5pejjb), "The world of today is different from that of one hundred years ago. We now have a much greater understanding of nature than our grandparents had. We have entered the atomic age, the electronic age, the nuclear age, the age of jet planes, television, and modern medicine and its wonder drugs. For the good of our health, we should also recognize that this is the age of vitamins."

Going further, Pauling asserts, "The discovery of vitamins during the first third of the twentieth century and the recognition that they are essential elements of a healthy diet was one of the most important contributions to health ever made. Of equal importance was the recognition, about twenty years ago, that the optimum intakes of several of the vitamins, far larger than the usually recommended intakes, lead to further improvement in health, greater protection against many diseases, and enhanced effectiveness in the therapy of diseases. The potency of vitamin C and other vitamins is explained by the new understanding that they function principally by strengthening the natural protective mechanisms of the body, especially the immune system."

Beginning back in the 1970's, the medical and pharmaceutical "establishment" took a dim view – and still do – of Linus Pauling's work. Here was this brilliant scientist explaining how the body functions – one cell at a time. When he then turned his attention to heart disease, he was talking about the curative powers of *inexpensive vitamins*. He was a threat to their line of reasoning, and to their profits.

The war for our hearts, minds and wallets was on. It was this genius altruist against the money and powerful influence of Big Pharma and the American Medical Association. We, the patients, have not stood much of a chance.

On one side stands the mighty conventional "Lipid Theory" of heart disease. Big Pharma employs an arsenal of patented (and therefore expensive) synthetic chemicals including statin drugs – along with invasive procedures ranging from stents to bypass surgery – to combat a symptom – "the enemy" – cholesterol. You cannot escape their constant advertising claims in the media.

The "Unified Theory" of heart disease, created and patented by Pauling and German doctor Matthias Rath, MD (https://tinyurl.com/y9f5wy63), stands in opposition. It has neither advertising budget nor a legion of sales weasels. It sees cholesterol as a **vital friend** to our bodies. It looks to restore heart health (horror of horrors!) *without the use of drugs*. Its forces consist of a small army of believers – people like myself, who have been lucky enough to learn about it, practice it, and enjoy restored health because of it. Those photos of my arteries scattered throughout this book are, quite literally, living proof.

§

When you look at another human being – or even yourself in a mirror – you see another human being. Medical scientists like Pauling and Rath see a complex assemblage of about 100 trillion individual living cells. The cell is the smallest unit of life that is classified as a living thing. Cells are the building blocks for every organ in your body. Cells live, die and get replaced over and over again throughout your lifetime. And cells can get sick.

Pauling was intrigued by the possibility of keeping cells healthy as a way of improving human health. Rath has carried on Pauling's interest in this field, but has become the focus of establishment derision because on occasion he has over-reached. He attempted to cure AIDS (as Pauling himself had suggested) in South Africa, for instance, using vitamins in hopes of helping cells fight off the disease. His experiments did not seem to work, several people in the study group died, and Rath and his program were banned. Like Pauling, too, he has been derided everywhere Big Pharma has influence, including the page about him in Wikipedia (https://tinyurl. com/ydcqa6y3). His supporters are fighting back with articles such as one attacking the legitimacy of Wikipedia itself (http:// tinyurl.com/ponzgvw).

Meanwhile, back to heart disease.

Using data they got from literally hundreds of published research papers by world-class scientists (MDs and PhDs), Pauling and Rath observed a curative link between cardio-vascular disease and vitamin C. They would build on this knowledge to form their "Unified Theory of Human Cardiovas-cular Disease." The Unified Theory describes how the human body exactly regulates blood concentrations of cholesterol; it offers a compelling argument that, with proper nutrition (and not drugs) cardiovascular disease can be prevented and even reversed.

Healthy cells, both Pauling and Rath reasoned, could better fight off disease and resist organ fatigue. Pauling was particularly interested in the role vitamin C plays in the health of cells. In his 1970 book, *Vitamin C and the Common Cold* (https://tinyurl.com/ycf3ytwb), Pauling advanced the idea that major doses of vitamin C could benefit human health. He was beginning to formulate his concept that many human illnesses could be traced back to a hidden, low-level version of scurvy.

Quoting from, Wikipedia (https://tinyurl.com/mnh7shg), "Scurvy is a disease resulting from a deficiency of vitamin C, which is required for the synthesis of collagen in humans. … Scurvy often presents itself initially as symptoms of malaise and lethargy, followed by formation of spots on the skin, spongy gums, and bleeding from the mucous membranes. Spots are most abundant on the thighs and legs, and a person with the ailment looks pale, feels depressed, and is partially immobilized. As scurvy advances, there can be open, suppurating wounds, loss of teeth, jaundice, fever, neuropathy and death."

In *How to Live Longer and Feel Better*, Pauling recalls the history of scurvy, once considered a plague of mankind. Between July 9, 1497 and May 30, 1498, for instance, explorer Vasco da Gama lost 100 of his 160-man crew to the disease. In 1577 a Spanish galleon was discovered adrift, its entire crew killed by scurvy. In 1741, Pauling reports, a British squadron of six ships lost half its sailors, dead from scurvy. Many California Gold Rush miners died of scurvy, too.

The British, Pauling says, were first to realize that fresh fruits and vegetables could prevent or reduce this disease. Keeping fruits or vegetables from spoiling on long sea voyages, though, was a problem, until they hit on lemons and limes. Eventually, all British sailors were issued daily rations of fresh lime juice. They became known as "Limeys," a label that would stick through the ages.

It would be years later, though, before research would reveal the reason lime juice worked. It contained a high concentration of ascorbic acid (vitamin C).

Another incident Pauling recalls riveted his attention on invisible forms of low-level scurvy … and the curative powers of vitamin C to strengthen blood vessels throughout the body:

"E. Cheraskin, W.M. Ringsdorf, Jr., and E.L. Sisley in their book, *The Vitamin C Connection* (1983) (https://tinyurl.com/y9gpph56)," Pauling reports, "recount the story of a forty-eight-year-old woman in California who came to the hospital because of pain, indigestion, and swelling of the abdomen. Over a period of four years she had six surgical operations. Each time the abdomen was found to be full of blood. In the effort to prevent the recurrent bleeding, her ovaries, uterus, appendix, spleen and part of the small intestine were removed. Finally, after four years, a doctor asked her what she ate and found that her diet contained essentially no fruits or vegetables and that she took no supplementary vitamins. She was getting a little vitamin C in her food, enough to keep her from dying of scurvy but not a sufficient amount to keep her blood vessels strong enough to prevent internal bleeding;. Her blood level of vitamin C was only 0.06 mg per deciliter. When she was put on 1000 mg of vitamin C per day she regained normal health, qualified, however, by the surgery she had endured."

Without sufficient vitamin C, her blood vessels grew weak and leaked blood into her abdomen. With sufficient vitamin C, her blood vessels grew stronger and stopped leaking. Hmmmm. Hold that thought.

§

Pauling and Rath looked at studies going back decades, and conducted research of their own. Their findings are in conflict with what we have been programmed to believe.

As naturopath and Pauling advocate/chronicler Owen R. Fonorow recalls on his website (https://tinyurl.com/ycdzvpr9), "The theory that Cardiovascular Disease (CVD) is related to a deficiency of vitamin C was first proposed by the Canadian physician G. C. Willis in 1953. He found that atherosclerotic plaques form over vitamin-C-starved vascular tissues in both guinea pigs and human beings. In 1989, after the discoveries of the Lp(a) cholesterol molecule (*circa* 1964) and its lysine binding sites (*circa* 1987), Linus Pauling and his associate Matthias Rath formulated a unified theory of heart disease and invented a cure."

Willis was the first to suggest that heart arteries were damaged by high blood pressures within those arteries (much higher than the blood pressure in your arms) combined with mechanical stress caused by the constantly pounding heart beat. Pauling and Rath studied Willis' observation that plaque does not form randomly throughout the body. For example, in a heart bypass, veins from the leg are used, in part at least, because they contain no plaque.

There was also this curiosity to consider. Wouldn't you think, if plaque build-up were caused by cholesterol particles floating in the blood, that the tiniest blood vessels would be the first to plug up? Wouldn't large vessels hosting a torrent of blood, such as carotid arteries in the neck and coronary arteries, flush away those particles before they could build up, and wouldn't those vessels be the last to develop blockages? But the opposite is generally true.

Based on the work of Willis and others, Pauling and Rath concluded that arteries in human hearts are deprived of adequate vitamin C. So, the root cause of coronary artery disease, they determined, is artery weakness, "localized scurvy," brought on by lack of enough vitamin C reaching the heart. In their weakened condition, coronary arteries yield to high pressures and a constantly pounding pulse; and lesions (cracks) then develop.

"Why only humans and not other creatures?" they wondered. Their answer is that almost all mammals, (except for guinea pigs, fruit bats, monkeys and humans) produce vitamin C naturally by enzymatic conversion of blood sugar to ascorbate, the type of vitamin C that is continually produced in the liver of most animals. It has been reported, for instance, that a 160-pound goat creates in its body about 13,000 milligrams of vitamin C per day.

According to the online publication, Human Gene Therapy (http://tinyurl.com/nra66an) genetic research is under way that may someday lead to humans regaining the ability to create their own vitamin C. Researchers in 2008 successfully restored the ability to do just that in a strain of lab mice that had been bred to no longer produce its own vitamin C. In less than 23 days, gene therapy was so effective that vitamin C levels in the defective mice were restored to those of normal mice who naturally make their own vitamin C.

So, long term, perhaps we will make enough of our own vitamin C to ward off heart disease, stroke and other organ failure. Keeping our individual cells healthy, as Pauling and Rath suggest, just might be the Holy Grail of longevity, the real "Fountain of Youth."

For now, though, the solution Pauling and Rath hit upon to strengthen heart arteries was daily intake of massive doses of vitamin C.

§

Meanwhile, Pauling and Rath wondered, suppose you do restore strength to heart arteries, then what do you do to clean out existing plaque formations?

That is when they turned their attention to the chemical make up of the gummy substance that builds up in weakened arteries. What was it? And, why was it there?

Beginning during the Korean War, scientists began examining the artery walls of deceased GI's and of other people who died of coronary artery disease. They were looking for LDL, the "bad" form of cholesterol, and by golly, they found it. For decades it was settled science that plaque build up in artery walls consisted mainly of LDL.

But in the late 80's Dr. Rath, working with researchers U. Beisiegel, A. Niendorf, K. Wolf, and T. Reblin, pursued work begun by Berg and others, and began looking at another substance found in plaque. It was the sticky cousin of LDL, another form of lipoprotein identified as Lipoprotein (a), referred to as Lp(a) (http://tinyurl.com/oc9x63j).

Lp(a), they concluded, was like the fireman rushing to the scene of a fire. Except, the body uses Lp(a) to patch up those lesions (cracks) that develop in arteries weakened by a lack of sufficient vitamin C. Lp(a), they theorized, rushes to the rescue. Its sticky surfaces plug the crack on one side, and grab any passing LDL on the other to help build a scab over the site of the wound.

Lp(a) starts with a highly-oxidized variety of LDL that attaches itself to a specific protein (Apo A). Together, they become Lipoprotein A or Lp(a). These really sticky molecules of Lp(a) seemed to be the glue in a process that patches arteries from the inside. It could also be implicated in how blood clots form.

2018 Update. Logically, Big Pharma – continuing to protect its cash cow, statin drugs – has come up with its newest enemy, Lp(a). Denying its essential role observed by Pauling, Rath and others, the campaign is on to chemically rid your body of this *dangerous substance.* Enter the Lipo-protein a Foundation (https://tinyurl.com/ybw27kla). So, here we go again. How can supposedly intelligent researchers be so dumb?

Pairing Pauling's decades of interest in vitamin C with Rath's work involving Lp(a) was a seminal event. Pauling brought the artery-healing theory of vitamin C therapy. With Rath came the idea that something other than LDL was plugging up heart arteries. That "something," he and his colleagues concluded, was Lp(a).

Others, too, were studying Lp(a). As early as 1986 the American Heart Association's very own journal, *Circulation*, was reporting the findings of another group: They reported Lp(a) was associated with CAD (coronary artery disease) in women of *all* ages. It was a factor, too, in men younger than 55. The apparent threshold for coronary risk was Lp(a) concentrations of approximately 10 to 13 mg/dl. And Lp(a) **appeared to be a major coronary risk factor** in the white patients studied, with a significance approaching that of the level of LDL or HDL cholesterol. *Circulation* 74, No. 4, 758-765, 1986 (http://tinyurl.com/ndmgbnt). (Emphasis mine)

Drug companies remain unimpressed. They have continued to focus attention (yours, mine, and our doctors) on "bad"

LDL and "good" HDL. And now they have added Lp(a) – as a cause rather than a symptom.

I call this the Carl Malden analogy. In the 1970s and '80s actor Carl Malden appeared in many commercials for American Express Travelers Checks. In every one of them Malden appeared on camera right after someone's money had been stolen – to proclaim this would not have happened had they carried Travelers Checks.

Wags opined it was quite suspicious that Malden appeared at the scene of all those crimes. The same might be said today for Lp(a) and LDL.

§

But why were these plaque blockages forming in the first place, and what did they have to do with weakened arteries? Pauling and Rath set about finding out.

To make a long story short, they knew, from the research of others, that weakened arteries were likely to develop cracks. "Lesions" is the term doctors use. Picture a tubeless tire with a small puncture. Like a blow-out patch on the inside of that tire, plaque builds up over a lesion to prevent an arterial blow-out. In other words, plaque is a *symptom* of heart disease, but not the cause.

So, perhaps rather than being a bad thing – to be compressed against artery walls with a balloon, or held in place with a stent, or removed with lasers or a type of "Roto-Rooter" – plaque is saving lives every day. Until, that is, it breaks loose or otherwise blocks a vital artery.

The twin goals, then, for Pauling and Rath, were to a) strengthen heart arteries with massive doses of vitamin C to prevent the need for the body to build up plaque, and b) to clear those restored arteries safely of existing plaque to prevent it from causing future heart attacks.

They knew how to strengthen arteries. But what to do about that gummy plaque buildup?

§

Coming back to Pauling's theory of using vitamin C to restore health to heart arteries, it is noteworthy that some heart specialists are now calling arthrosclerosis a "systemic disease." By that they mean it is necessary to treat all the heart's arteries, not just areas where plaque has built up.

In a New York Times article published March 21, 2004 (website: https://tinyurl.com/ou74ek6), a Dr. Waters of the University of California is quoted, talking about his 1999 research, "We were saying that atherosclerosis is a systemic disease. It occurs throughout all the coronary arteries. If you fix one segment, a year later it will be another segment that pops and gives you a heart attack, so systemic therapy … has the potential to do a lot more."

Of course the "systemic therapy" Waters had in mind was even greater use of "statins or antiplatelet drugs." Has your doctor yet recommended them for your children?

That Pauling and Rath were proposing vitamin C to strengthen arteries – and proposing a course of action to remove plaque build up everywhere in the body – was and remains medical heresy to this day. Yet, it makes so much sense.

Have your gums ever bled when you flossed your teeth? Have you ever had a nosebleed for no apparent reason? Have you ever had a wound that was slow to heal? If so, you may have had a deficiency of vitamin C in your system. Often – it would appear from Pauling and Rath's work – lack of vitamin C is overlooked when a person develops a chronic condition (which adds stress to the body and further depletes already inadequate ascorbate stores). Tell-tale symptoms of scurvy may appear but the correct diagnosis may be missed and instead called some chronic disease (i.e., poor wound healing in diabetics, hemorrhages in diseases like Crohn's and ulcerative colitis, etc.).

§

Most of us are walking around suffering from what I would call *"lack-of-adequate-vitamin C disease,"* but our doctors – encouraged by the pharmaceutical industry – just keep treating our *symptoms.* More on this in Chapters 8 and 9.

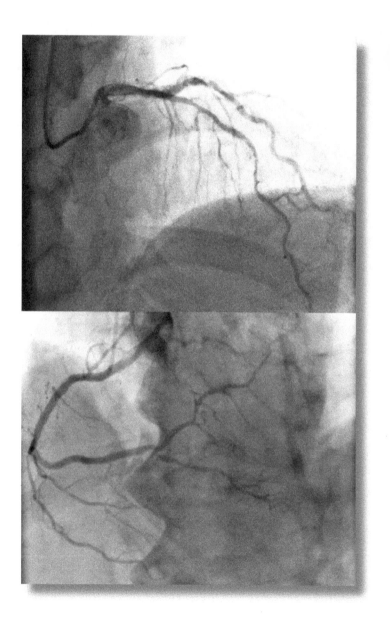

CHAPTER FIVE

WHY THE "PAULING/RATH PROTOCOL" WORKS

READER CAUTION: THIS IS THE TECHNICAL STUFF. CINCH UP THINKING CAPS NOW.

Pauling was big on something called collagen.

Now, in Hollywood, collagen injections are popular, mostly to inflate lips and to fill wrinkles, lines and scars on the face and sometimes the neck, back and chest. *Collagen* means, "glue producer" (kola = glue in Greek) – because glue has been made for centuries by boiling animal sinew and hooves. The gelatin in Jell-O comes from the *collagen* in cow or pig bones, hooves, and connective tissues.

But Pauling was focused on the collagen that forms naturally, inside of you. In fact collagen is the most abundant protein in your body. It forms into fibers which are stronger than iron wire of comparable size. These fibers provide strength and stability to all body tissues, including your arteries.

And collagen formation requires large amounts of vitamin C.

Here is a transcript of poor old, doddering imbecile Linus Pauling (as Big Pharma portrayed him) from that 1994 video (https://tinyurl.com/yb2dpjbm) created just prior to his death:

"Collagen is made in rather large amounts in human bodies and in the bodies of other mammals. It strengthens the blood vessels and the skin, and the muscles, and the bones, and the teeth. A very important substance. You can't make collagen without using up vitamin C. Collagen is made from another protein, 'procollagen,' by hydroxlilating *Lys-Ile* and Pro-Ile residues in the procollagen and converting them into hydroxi-Lys-Ile and hydroxi-Pro-Ile residues. With every hydroxyl group that is introduced, one ascorbate ion (one molecule of vitamin C) is used up. Most animals manufacture their own vitamin C in their livers, and they manufacture it in such large amounts that their blood vessels and other tissues are stronger than those of human beings and do not develop the sort of lesions that result in overt cardiovascular disease such as humans get."

Oh, yes, obviously doddering and demented, wasn't he? But that's what Big Pharma claimed!

Expanding on that Pauling quote, collagen is the most abundant protein in the body. While literally a fiber, collagen acts like a "glue," one that holds our cells together. Collagen is actually the body's preferred repair substance – for closing wounds, healing blood vessels, or helping the skin look its best.

The collagen fiber looks like a 3-strand rope. It contains a strand of L-glycine molecules, a strand of L-proline molecules, and a strand of L-lysine molecules. Under a powerful microscope, these strands can be seen twisted around each other. They do, in fact, look like a rope. When an injury happens and the collagen fiber breaks, the frayed ends dangle exactly like a damaged rope.

As Pauling explained in scientific language, above, if enough ascorbate (vitamin C) is available, the amino acid molecules at the broken ends are "hydroxylated." That means the "end" molecules of L-glycine, lysine and proline are chemically changed. They become L-hydroxyglycine, L-hydroxylysine and L-hydroxyproline.

This chemical process allows those frayed ends to be spliced back together (much like boatswain's mates who worked for me in the Navy would splice rope). As Pauling explained, "With every hydroxyl group that is introduced, one ascorbate ion (one molecule of vitamin C) is used up." In other words, vitamin C is absolutely essential for the production and repair of collagen, *and vitamin C is destroyed during the process.* That is why consuming large amounts of vitamin C – to replace vitamin C destroyed in this process – is key to healing damaged arteries.

As we saw in Chapter Four, the first part of the Pauling Protocol is consumption of massive amounts of vitamin C. The vitamin C nourishes collagen in our trillions of cells and restores health to damaged blood vessels. Because your body flushes it from your system so quickly, the only way to flood heart vessels with enough vitamin C to keep them healthy is to take large doses, preferably at least three times each day.

As for those three key amino acids, L-glycine is the least complex and, in general, the body always makes enough. L-lysine and L-proline, though, are not always in sufficient supply. So you need to take L-lysine and L-proline supplements, along with vitamin C, to ensure adequate collagen repair.

§

While Pauling was interested in collagen and the health of heart arteries, Rath was looking at the nature of that "blowout patch," the build up of plaque inside weakened arteries. If arteries could be restored to health, how could the plaque be prevented from breaking loose, possibly to cause a fatal heart attack?

The answer was to remove the plaque; but how?

All lipoproteins are molecules made of proteins and fat. They carry cholesterol and other necessary substances through the blood. While nearly everyone else was looking at LDL and HDL, Rath and his colleagues had been studying Lp(a).

Lipoprotein (a) is a type of cholesterol carrier found *only* in species that *do not* produce their own vitamin C. When there is not enough vitamin C circulating in your arteries to keep you healthy, your body looks to Lp(a) to patch damaged blood vessels and keep you from dying of internal hemorrhage. So, surprising to most of us, the LDL on which the entire statin industry is based is *not* the main culprit.

Sticky Lp(a) particles circulate in your blood. When a blood vessel wall is damaged, they are attracted to those frayed collagen "ropes" we talked about earlier. In particular, they bond with the lysine fragments. As Lp(a) begins to coat your broken lysine strands, free lysine in the blood is drawn to the Lp(a). This process continues as lysine and Lp(a) are both drawn from your blood to build ever-larger amounts of plaque. Gradually this "blow out patch" grows in thickness. Over time, it can reduce the inner diameter of an artery and restrict its capacity to carry blood. In the worst case, you have a heart attack and die.

A report from Berkeley HeartLab, a wholly-owned subsidiary of Quest Diagnostics, finds the following about Lp(a): "Lipoprotein(a) was first described in 1963 and subsequently ascribed a role as a cardiovascular risk factor. Lp(a) is a plasma lipoprotein, produced in the liver, very similar in structure and density to LDL, having a cholesterol-rich triglyceride (TG) core encapsulated by a layer of phospholipids and free cholesterol. Like all non-high density lipoprotein (non-HDL) particles, every Lp(a) has a single molecule of apolipoprotein B (apoB) attached to the surface. Similar to LDL particles, both the lipid core and the attached apoB in Lp(a) are atherogenic."

(Author's comment: In layman's terms, atherogenic means "hardening of the arteries.")

2018 Update. Berkeley HeartLab is defunct. Quest Diagnostics bought them, but was recently fined $6 million because Berkeley had been bribing doctors and patients. Searches for

Berkeley now lead to web pages like this: https://tinyurl.com/y849868o.

§

If you waded through all that, you figured out that Lp(a) is like LDL, *yet different*. And that difference is what Rath and Pauling were able to exploit.

They went looking for something that could circulate in the blood and both neutralize and remove Lp(a) after arteries had been restored to health by vitamin C. They found just that in L-Lyzine. That's right. Not only does L-Lyzine play a role in repairing collagen and heart arteries, but molecules of this substance circulating in your blood are also able to bond with a receptor on the surface of the Lp(a) molecule – no longer needed for that "blow out patch" – and gradually drag it away to the liver to be flushed from your system.

§

Later, Rath and Pauling found that L-Proline is equal to, or even better than L-Lyzine in its ability to remove Lp(a). L-proline is a unique amino acid. It prefers to be in oil rather than water. L-proline is thus lipophilic as opposed to L-lysine, which prefers water and is hydrophilic.

Lp(a) is a combination of a water-loving protein (apo a) and oily cholesterol. Pauling and Rath theorized that lipophilic L-proline would block receptors on the oily portion of Lp(a). When they added L-proline to their vitamin C and L-lysine solution, the effects were astounding. Blockages completely disappeared.

§

So, here's the deal in a nutshell. Vitamin C is sacrificed to repair your dangling lysine and proline strands of collagen. This process prevents and/or repairs artery damage. With your artery health restored, there are no longer any frayed lysine and proline strands in vessel walls. There is no longer a "fit" for the Lp(a)'s receptor sites. Gradually, Lp(a) particles (or plaque patches) start to erode from the now-healthy artery walls.

Massive doses of vitamin C promote healthy heart arteries. Large doses of L-Lyzine and L-Proline clean up the mess left behind (arterial plaque), and sweep the arteries clean. Maintenance levels of these three over-the-counter, inexpensive supplements can keep things that way. Again, reference those photos of my arteries scattered throughout this book. They are, quite literally, living proof.

§

To add further emphasis to the vitamin C and Lysine theory, there is this. Pauling and Rath were granted yet another U.S. patent (# 5230996) (https://tinyurl.com/yayupkvz) for a solution containing vitamin C and L-lysine, this one *to remove plaques from donor organs* prior to transplant surgery. (Emphasis mine)

When a transplanted organ is in place, blood must quickly disperse through the new organ or its tissue will soon die.

Bathing transplanted organs in this vitamin C-lysine solution before implantation *removed plaques in major vessels* and greatly improved transplantation outcomes. Pretty impressive for vitamin C and a lowly amino acid, don't you think? Newer, more effective, organ cleansing methods have since taken the place of Pauling and Rath's discovery, but it remains evidence of the power of vitamin C and L-Lysine (now supplemented with L-Proline) to restore health to heart arteries.

Oh, how I wish I had paid better attention in high school science and biology classes. I might have been able to bore you with even greater details on how all this works.

Tossing a bone to the scientists among us ...

Vitamin C Chemical Structure
Source: New World Encyclopedia
https://tinyurl.com/y9mf9rqr

L-Lysine Chemical Structure
Source: About.com Chemistry

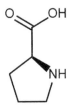

(http://tinyurl.com/od35yha)
L-Proline Chemical Structure
Source: PubChem
https://tinyurl.com/y8jacxz4

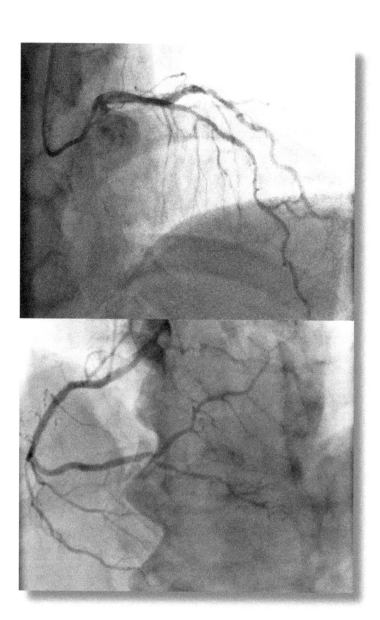

CHAPTER SIX

WHAT PAULING AND OTHERS HAVE SUGGESTED ADDING TO THE PROTOCOL

Remember, Pauling and Rath's "Unified Theory" borrows from the naturopathy branch of medicine – unlike its opposite, Big Pharma's "Lipid Theory," which treats diseases and symptoms with patentable (profitable) synthetic chemicals, such as statin drugs.

And remember, too, Pauling was focused on restoring health to each of the trillions of individual living cells that make up our bodies. He reasoned you can not do that – in most instances – simply with chemicals and drugs.

Throughout the ages and up until the early 1900's, our bodies depended on natural substances for their health. All wild animals still do. Wild animals don't get injections. They don't pop pills. Mostly, they are able to get all the nutrition they need to remain healthy from the food they eat.

But have you looked at the food labels in you cupboards and refrigerator lately? "Natural" is not us. More and more, our systems are bathed in preservatives, flavor enhancers and other unnatural substances to "improve" their taste and shelf life. We get more salt in a bowl of soup than we need in an entire day. Essential vitamins and minerals are cooked out of processed foods. Worries are mounting that the beef, pork and poultry we consume are tainted with growth enhancers, and that antibiotics given to animals raised for food are causing the viruses that attack us to mutate into forms less responsive to antibiotics for people. It has even been suggested that little girls are coming of age sooner these days due to growth hormones in the meat they consume.

In short, cells in every part of our bodies are under siege every day from many of the foods we eat and from chemicals older generations never experienced. While vitamin C is essential to the collagen that we need for healthy cells – to coin a phrase – man cannot live on amino acid alone. Nor can we rely simply on the foods we eat.

Realizing this, Pauling added to his three basic heart ingredients – massive doses of vitamin C, L-Lysine and L-Proline – a list of other vitamins and minerals he *recommends* for healthy bones, muscles, brains and teeth.

Following is a summary of Pauling's earlier recommended supplementation from his 1986 book, How to Live Longer and Feel Better, as that list appears on the Cancer Survival website (https://tinyurl.com/y7eeydg6)

1. Take vitamin C every day, 6 grams (g) to 18 g (6,000 to 1,800 milligrams [mg]) or more. Do not miss a single day.
2. Take vitamin E every day, 400 IU, 800 IU, or 1600 IU.
3. Take one or more Super-B tablets every day, to provide good amounts of the B vitamins.
4. Take a 25,000 IU vitamin A or a 15 mg, beta-carotene tablet every day.
5. Take a mineral supplement every day, such as one tablet of the Bronson Vitamin-Mineral Formula.
6. Keep your intake of ordinary sugar (sucrose, raw sugar, brown sugar, honey) to 50 pounds per year, which is half the present US average. Do not add sugar to tea or coffee. Do not eat high-sugar foods. Avoid sweet desserts. Do not drink soft drinks.
7. Except for avoiding sugar, eat what you like-but not too much of any one food. Eggs and meat are good foods. Also, you should eat some vegetables and fruits. Do not eat so much food as to become obese.
8. Drink plenty of water every day.
9. Keep active; take some exercise. Do not at any time exert yourself physically to an extent far beyond what you are accustomed to.
10. Drink alcoholic beverages only in moderation.
11. DO NOT SMOKE CIGARETTES.
12. Avoid stress. Work at a job that you like. Be happy with your family.

Nutritionist and health consultant Jonathan Campbell (https://tinyurl.com/y8k4urvf), in his 2005 booklet entitled "The End of Cardiovascular Disease," updated Pauling's 1986 list by suggesting the following additional supplements for good health.

Recommended Supplement	Recovery Mode	Maintenance Mode
Magnesium glycinate (or other magnesium-amino acid chelate)	Calcium 1,000 mg Magnesium 500 mg twice daily	Calcium 500 mg Magnesium 250 mg twice daily
Acetyl-L-Carnitine	500 mg. twice daily	500 mg. twice daily
Vitamin E	400 IU daily	400 IU daily
Beta carotene (vitamin A source)	20,000 IU daily in two doses	20,000 IU daily in two doses
Omega-3 (n-3) fatty acids	Pharmaceutical Grade Fish Oil 2000 mg EPA/1000 mg DHA daily	Pharmaceutical Grade Fish Oil 2000 mg EPA/1000 mg DHA daily
Coenzyme Q10	50-100 mg 3 times daily with meals	50-100 mg 3 times daily with meals
Glucosamine	1,000 mg twice daily	1,000 mg twice daily
Methylsulfonylmethane (MSM)	1,000 mg twice daily	1,000 mg twice daily
N-acetylcysteine	500 mg twice daily	

Recommended Supplement	Recovery Mode	Maintenance Mode
Zinc	40-50 mg total	30 mg daily
Potassium Citrate	500 mg three times daily	500 mg three times daily
High-dosage Multi-Vitamin/Mineral Complex	Daily	Daily
Grapeseed Extract	150-300 mg daily	150-300 mg daily
Alpha Lipoic Acid	500 mg twice daily	500 mg twice daily
Chlorella	2,500 mg three times daily	2,500 mg three times daily
Lecithin granules	2 tblspns daily	
Organic Flaxseed Oil	2 tblspns daily	2 tblspns daily
Water	2 Quarts daily	2 Quarts daily
Soy Protein Drink	1/2 Scoop X3	1/2 Scoop X3
Copper	2 mg daily	2 mg daily

Others, too, have expanded on Pauling's list of suggested supplements for a healthy heart and body. For example, Thomas E. Levy, MD, JD (https://tinyurl.com/y7nzxk7s), in his book, *Stop America's #1 Killer* (https://tinyurl.com/yccprp8q), recommends the following additional items:

Recommended Supplement	Daily Intake
L-arginine	500 to 1,500 mg daily
Menatetrenone (vitamin K2)	3 to 9 mg daily
Cholecalciferol (vitamin D3)	400 to 1,000 IU daily
L-carnosine	200 to 1,000 mg daily
Thiamine (vitamin B1)	50 to 500 mg daily
Pyridoxine (vitamin B6)	25 to 100 mg daily
Riboflavin (vitamin B2)	5 to 15 mg daily
Pantothenic acid (vitamin B5)	10 to 15 mg daily
Biotin (vitamin B7)	300 to 500 micrograms daily
Folic acid (vitamin B9)	400 to 500 micrograms daily
Cobalamin (vitamin B12)	15 to 20 micrograms daily
Niacin (vitamin B3)	20 to 25 mg daily
Superoxide dismutase (SOD)	100 to 400 mg daily
Chondroitin sulfate C (chondroitin 6-sulfate)	500 to 1,500 mg daily
Glutathione	500 to 1,500 mg daily
Chromium	100 to 200 micrograms daily
Manganese	'0.5 to 1.0 mg daily
Selenium	100 to 200 micrograms daily
Vanadium	10 to 50 micrograms daily
Indium	25 to 50 micrograms daily
Boron	15 to 20 micrograms daily

§

Beyond vitamin C, L-Lysine, L-Proline, plus the basic list recommended by Linus Pauling, I recommend you research according to your own needs. The above discussion is presented simply to make you aware that many others are continuing to add to the work of Pauling and Rath.

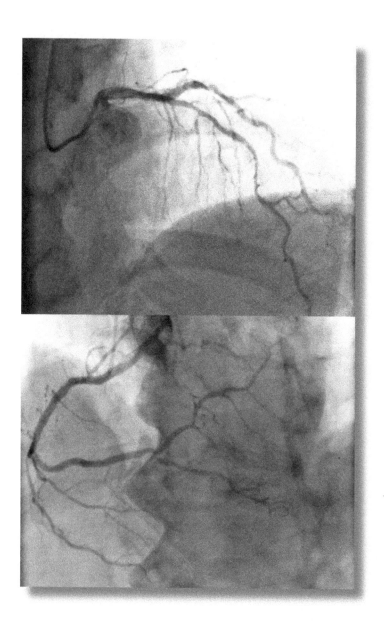

CHAPTER SEVEN

BUT WHAT ABOUT CHOLESTEROL? AND WHAT DO I EAT NOW?

"Why do you think an egg yolk is full of cholesterol? Because it takes a lot of cholesterol to build a healthy chicken. It also takes a hell of a lot to build and maintain a healthy human being. In fact, cholesterol is so vital that almost all cells can manufacture cholesterol; one of the key functions of the liver is to synthesize cholesterol. It's vital for the proper functioning of the brain and it's the building block for most sex hormones."
—Malcolm Kendrick, MD (MbChB MRCGP)
peer-reviewer for the British Medical Journal, and member of the International Network of Cholesterol Skeptics (Thincs), from his 2007 article, "Have we been conned about cholesterol?" published in the U.K. Daily Mail On Line (http://tinyurl.com/5bvjf4)

B ack a generation or two, it used to be really something when you heard "the rabbit died." Depending on the circumstances, it could mean great joy. At other times, women could become hysterical. Grown men cried. A dead rabbit meant some woman was pregnant.

Animal testing was the norm back then, and rabbits were perhaps more guinea pigs than Guinea Pigs. So, it wasn't surprising, in 1956, when some bozos in white lab coats in South Africa force fed massive quantities of cholesterol to bunnies and a surprising number of the poor little rabbits died.

Here is part of the cover page of their report as it appears on the Internet (http://tinyurl.com/oebchp2):

Brit. J. Haemat., 1957, 3, 366.

Blood Coagulation Abnormalities Produced by Feeding Cholesterol to Rabbits

C. MERSKEY

Department of Medicine,* University of Cape Town, South Africa

ABNORMALITIES of blood coagulation have been observed in cholesterol-fed rabbits (Merskey, Sapeika, Uys and Bronte-Stewart, 1956). Rabbits which received cholesterol and phenindione (phenylindanedione, P.I.D., Dindevan) were noted to have a higher mortality (mainly from haemorrhage) than rabbits fed cholesterol without phenindione. Even without phenindione, rabbits receiving cholesterol developed a prolonged coagulation time and excessive amounts of residual prothrombin remained in the serum after coagulation. In general this defect developed as the serum cholesterol rose and there was correlation between elevation of the serum cholesterol and the development of the coagulation defect. In this paper the fully-developed coagulation abnormalities of the cholesterol-fed rabbits are described.

There you have it. Rabbits – who produce their own vitamin C and seldom develop heart disease – got saturated with gooey, sticky cholesterol that their bodies had no use for, and their arteries clogged up. It happened because their normal vegetarian diet was taken away, and they were forced to survive on eggs and other foods unnatural to rabbits.

When the cholesterol diet was withdrawn, the surviving bunnies had miraculous recoveries. The conclusion? Cholesterol kills *people*. And, presto! A new fake "disease" was invented, and the race was on to find a "cure."

That questionable beginning launched the "Lipid Theory" of heart disease. It speculates that harmful levels of a waxy substance (cholesterol) circulate in your blood. You need the "good" kind (HDL), but the "bad" kind (LDL) is just waiting for the opportunity to stick itself to otherwise healthy blood vessels and gum them up. For some unexplained reason, LDL only does this in larger arteries (carotid, cardiovascular), where you might expect torrents of blood under high pressure would sweep it away. It seldom, if ever, blocks smaller arteries or veins. Go figure.

Here's the crash course. Your liver produces "lipoproteins" (i.e., lipids and proteins) which then circulate in your blood. Lipids are naturally occurring molecules that include fats; waxes; sterols; fat-soluble vitamins such as A, D, E and K; monoglycerides, diglycerides, and other substances.

Lipoproteins can be further defined as various types of cholesterol, triglycerides, fatty acids, and phospholipids, among others. There's an industry of folks who measure and quantify these things in your blood – and a much bigger, and very profitable, industry dedicated to manipulating their levels in your bloodstream.

In reality, your lipids are like military Meals Ready to Eat, carried by your blood stream to nourish cell membranes everywhere in your body. Everywhere. It's a closed loop, with LDL carrying fresh supplies to your cells, and HDL bringing waste products back to your liver (http://tinyurl.com/bryr5q5).

Yet, the "Lipid Theory" tries to distinguish between "good" (HDL) and "bad" (LDL) cholesterol. It seeks to increase the former and diminish the latter.

Here's the problem. There is no evidence that the levels of these substances in your blood – or attempts at controlling them, for that matter – will increase (or decrease) your chances of dying from coronary artery disease.

One of my favorite people in the great cholesterol debate is the Scottish M.D., Malcolm Kendrick, author of *The Great Cholesterol Con* (https://tinyurl.com/y83xok6a) (see the quote from him that opened this chapter). He's a favorite because he took the time to analyze studies conducted by the World Health Organization (WHO) (Web link: http://tinyurl.com/nfe7c7r).

In its global MONICA (Multinational MONItoring of trends and determinants in CArdiovascular disease) Project, WHO studied cholesterol levels in populations around the world. This was a major project, collecting decades of research from scientists in dozens of countries. The MONICA scientists also analyzed deaths by heart attack in a couple dozen countries. As luck would have it, fifteen countries or groups of people ended up in both reports.

Kendrick's approach was ingenious. He made a line graph of average cholesterol levels in those fifteen countries. Next he superimposed a second line graph over the first. This one, also from MONICA, studied "Death Rates from Heart Disease in Males Aged 35 – 74" *in those very same countries.* **You can see the results on the back cover of this book.**

Famously, lines from those two charts do not match. Not even close. Australian Aborigines have among the highest death rates from heart disease in the world. Yet, their cholesterol levels are by far the lowest among the fifteen regions studied. And Switzerland, with the highest blood cholesterol levels, has among the very lowest death rates from heart disease. France, too, in what has become known as "the French Paradox" – because the French delight in cheeses and creams is supposed to ramp up heart disease there but it does not.

There is a very short YouTube video of Dr. Kendrick with his graph. If you missed the link above, it is truly eye opening. You should take one minute to view it here: http://tinyurl.com/nfe7c7r

If it were not deadly serious, it would be funny, but here is a YouTube cartoon that adds perspective to Kendrick's work: http://tinyurl.com/q5n3ony.

§

So, besides (supposedly) gumming up arteries, what does cholesterol do for you?

Let's talk about your brain. It weighs about three pounds. Like much of your body, 78 percent of it is water. Protein accounts for about eight percent. Carbohydrates and other substances make up about 4 percent. Between 10 and 12 percent is fat (remember that the next time someone calls you a fathead; they'll be semi-correct). Much of that fat (gasp) is cholesterol.

Your brain is made up of several types of cells with specific functions. One kind seemed to do very little, and was pretty much ignored until 2001. Then, a group of German and French researchers discovered these cells weren't lazy after all. Called "glial cells," they contain cholesterol – in fact, they make their own cholesterol. What they do with it is the amazing part. They use the stuff *to encourage your brain to manufacture synapses.*

Synapses, you may know, are the junctions or pathways that enable one cell to communicate with other cells. They're existence makes it possible for you to think and remember. When those researchers put glial nerve cells in a Petri dish and added plain cholesterol, synapses began forming before their eyes (well, under their microscopes, actually, but you get the picture).

Dr. Duane Graveline, MD (http://spacedoc.com/), was a former flight surgeon for the U.S. Air Force. He conducted space medicine research, was a NASA astronaut, practiced as a family physician for 20 years, and wrote eight books during his retirement. Yet, after six weeks on Lipitor, he experienced what is called "transient global amnesia" that lasted about six hours. During that time he could not remember most of his incredible life – nor recognize his wife and children. Concerned that Lipitor might have caused this, he stopped taking the drug despite his doctors' assurances.

A year later, when his doctors encouraged him to try Lipitor again, the amnesia soon returned, this time lasting 12 hours and sending him to the ER. Dr. Graveline's experiences led him to others who reported similar memory lapses after taking this drug. Further research resulted in his book, *Lipitor, Thief of Memory* (https://tinyurl.com/y94xp8g9).

In a subsequent book, *Statin Drugs Side Effects* (https://tinyurl.com/ydgouev7), Dr. Graveline cites a study by Muldoon, et al that found "100% of patients placed on statins showed measurable decrease in cognitive function after six months, whereas 100% of placebo treated control patients showed measurable increase in cognitive function during the same time period."

So, raise your hand if you want to deplete your brain of cholesterol. Didn't think so.

But, you know, that may have already happened. That is, if you have ever taken statin drugs. Statins do not discriminate. They don't just diminish cholesterol levels in your blood. They rob vital cholesterol from every organ in your body – including your brain.

I know this from personal experience. After all, I was on statin drugs a total of seventeen years. A few years ago I was so concerned about memory fog that I sought medical help. The good news was that my symptoms were not those of Alzheimer's. My IQ was still high, but my memory complaints were inexplicable.

For instance, I cannot remember a string of numbers longer than about four or five digits.

I enjoy watching NFL games on TV, but with few exceptions I cannot identify familiar faces of coaches and players on the sidelines. I enjoy watching the plays, but if I step away from the TV I have difficulty remembering the score or most of the previous plays.

Similarly, I enjoy watching the post-game shows with my wife, who is an avid fan. I like the replays and the interviews. Yet, again with few exceptions, don't ask me who was interviewed when the show ends.

This carries over to my writing.

I have been a professional writer most of my life – mostly press releases and short articles in various PR jobs. I ran my own consulting business for medical practices, a company called "Patient Relations," for about six years.

So, I know how to write. Keeping a train of thought going, though, has become difficult. In working on a chapter like this one, for instance, I can't tell you how many times I'll have to go back and read it from the beginning, so that I may gather my thoughts and continue.

Oddly, these lapses and losses of memory don't impact my ability to handle technical tasks. I can trouble shoot most computer glitches. Solutions come quickly to mind. I enjoy my Android smart phone, and have it loaded up with useful apps. Just don't ask me to name many of them without looking at the phone.

2018 Update: Despite taking several over-the-counter memory supplements, my memory issues have slowly gotten worse. I'm beginning to have "technical difficulties" dealing with technical difficulties. And thank God for modern spelling checkers, because my spelling has become atrocious.

§

Ever wonder who sets the target numbers for your HDL and LDL? Those numbers were adjusted downward again in 2004 – creating millions more patients who thus needed statin drugs. More than a few eyebrows were raised at the composition of the panel behind the *"Third Report of the Expert Panel on Detection, Evaluation, and Treatment of High Blood Cholesterol in Adults (Adult Treatment Panel III)* (https://tinyurl.com/yb4ft282).

Members of that board had more than a passing acquaintance with the companies that manufacture statin drugs, the same companies that stood to reap a fortune based on the panel's new numbers. Details about those relationships were revealed here:

P III UPDATE 2004: FINANCIAL DISCLOSURE

(**2018 Update NOTE:** The NIH has removed links to this data from the Internet. However, you can find that information recreated at https://tinyurl.com/ybhv734).

"Dr. Grundy has received honoraria from Merck, Pfizer, Sankyo, Bayer, Merck/Schering-Plough, Kos, Abbott, Bristol-Myers Squibb, and AstraZeneca; he has received research grants from Merck, Abbott, and Glaxo Smith Kline."

"Dr. Cleeman has no financial relationships to disclose."

"Dr. Bairey Merz has received lecture honoraria from Pfizer, Merck, and Kos; she has served as a consultant for Pfizer, Bayer, and EHC (Merck); she has received unrestricted institutional grants for Continuing Medical Education from Pfizer, Procter & Gamble, Novartis, Wyeth, AstraZeneca, and Bristol-Myers Squibb Medical Imaging; she has received a research grant from Merck; she has stock in Boston Scientific, IVAX, Eli Lilly, Medtronic, Johnson & Johnson, SCIPIE Insurance, ATS Medical, and Biosite."

"Dr. Brewer has received honoraria from AstraZeneca, Pfizer, Lipid Sciences, Merck, Merck/Schering-Plough, Fournier, Tularik, Esperion, and Novartis; he has served as a consultant for AstraZeneca, Pfizer, Lipid Sciences, Merck, Merck/Schering-Plough, Fournier, Tularik, Sankyo, and Novartis."

"Dr. Clark has received honoraria for educational presentations from Abbott, AstraZeneca, Bristol-Myers Squibb, Merck, and Pfizer; he has received grant/research support from Abbott, AstraZeneca, Bristol-Myers Squibb, Merck, and Pfizer."

"Dr. Hunninghake has received honoraria for consulting and speakers bureau from AstraZeneca, Merck, Merck/Schering-Plough, and Pfizer, and for consulting from Kos; he has received research grants from AstraZeneca, Bristol-Myers Squibb, Kos, Merck, Merck/Schering-Plough, Novartis, and Pfizer."

"Dr. Pasternak has served as a speaker for Pfizer, Merck, Merck/Schering-Plough, Takeda, Kos, BMS-Sanofi, and Novartis; he has served as a consultant for Merck, Merck/Schering-Plough, Sanofi, Pfizer Health Solutions, Johnson & Johnson-Merck, and AstraZeneca."

"Dr. Smith has received institutional research support from Merck; he has stock in Medtronic and Johnson & Johnson."

"Dr. Stone has received honoraria for educational lectures from Abbott, AstraZeneca, Bristol-Myers Squibb, Kos, Merck, Merck/

Schering-Plough, Novartis, Pfizer, Reliant, and Sankyo; he has served as a consultant for Abbott, Merck, Merck/Schering-Plough, Pfizer, and Reliant."

§

At least half of those who have succumbed to coronary artery disease have had HDL and LDL numbers in the "normal" range. Rather than consider that they are on the wrong track, members of these panels consistently conclude we need a "new normal." Their numbers go lower – incidentally creating millions of new consumers for their pharmaceutical mentors – yet deaths from coronary artery disease remain stubbornly unaffected. Odd, isn't it?

§

OK, so what does the Pauling/Rath diet consist of?

Pauling himself says to go back to a normal diet. Or, as Ben Franklin famously said, "All things in moderation."

If cholesterol is merely a boogey man, why play the no-cholesterol/low-cholesterol game? I have gone back to using real butter. I enjoy a flavorful, well-marbled steak from time to time. And deserts are no longer forbidden food.

Am I gorging myself? Absolutely not. My wife has other health issues, so I am eating healthier with her. We consume a lot of salad, in part because we enjoy it. Portions on our plates are smaller, and more in line with dietary recommendations. Where we once enjoyed a porterhouse or sirloin, each, we now share halves of one. We switch around between beef, chicken and pork (I might eat more fish, but she dislikes it, nor will she cook it).

From all those years of "watching my cholesterol," I have to admit I've developed one or two acquired tastes. Much as I like saltine crackers, I can't stand the regular ones anymore. They taste greasy and lackluster to me now, and I much prefer the fat-free kind. After giving up milk decades ago, I resorted to rice and soy products, but none really pleased me. Then, a few years ago, I discovered almond milk. I prefer it on my cereal now. Besides, I've read that cow's milk is designed to foster the growth of calves, and that no human over age six really needs that stuff.

But these are our personal peculiarities. The bottom line is, if you are following the Pauling/Rath protocol, enjoy what you want ... in moderation.

§

AND THERE IS THIS: "Researchers stopped a clinical trial when it failed to find any benefit from raising levels of HDL ('good') cholesterol with extended-release niacin. Adding the drug to a statin, a medication that lowers LDL ('bad') cholesterol, was expected to lead to a reduction in heart attacks and strokes. But there was no difference between those taking just a statin and people taking a statin plus niacin in how often heart disease developed. The study calls into question long-held beliefs about the benefits of raising levels of HDL cholesterol. But the findings may not apply to people with poorly controlled LDL or other risk factors for heart attack and stroke." *Source:* National Institutes of Health, May 26, 2011 (https://tinyurl.com/ycyb9bgb)

§

Add to the above a Reuters report, "**Low 'good' cholesterol doesn't cause heart attacks**," (http://tinyurl.com/y7yrspv8) referencing a study in the November 2011 *Journal of Clinical Endocrinology and Metabolism.* Although a first glance analysis of data on nearly 70,000 people in Denmark seemed to show a link between low levels of high-density lipoprotein (HDL) – the so-called "good" cholesterol – and raised heart attack risk, there was a nagging problem. In people with a gene mutation that lowers HDL, heart attack risk was not found to be higher at all.

That finding suggests something other than low HDL must be causing heart attacks. Or, as Reuters reported, "'Association itself doesn't mean causality,' said lead author Dr. Ruth Frikke-Schmidt, a consultant in the Department of Clinical Biochemistry at Rigshospitalet in Copenhagen." (November, 2012, Journal of Clinical Endocrinology and Metabolism: http://tinyurl.com/oh5stp9).

The results suggest that just having low HDL is not what raises the likelihood of a heart attack. "It's a total relook at what we thought was gospel," Dr. Christopher Cannon, professor of medicine at Harvard Medical School and editor of the American College of Cardiology's website, told Reuters.

NEW TO REPORT AS OF THIS 2018 UPDATE

Sadly, as noted in the IN MEMORIUM section below the table of contents for this edition, Dr. Duane Graveline passed away earlier this year. He attributed his decline and eventual death (chronicled at http://tinyurl.com/y8294xrd) to Lipitor. His final book, *The Dark Side of Statins* (https://tinyurl.com/yc5blx9d), was published after his death, in August, 2017. His own synopsis of the book appears here: https://tinyurl.com/yck99nr3

My own status, too, is declining. Like him, I attribute this to my 17 years on statin drugs. Like his early symptoms, too, I have developed *non-diabetic* peripheral neuropathy in both feet which has progressed to my ankles.

More concerning has been my progressive loss of memory. Now age 76, I find I have less and less recall of recent events; like mistakenly re-ordering an item I had purchased just a couple weeks prior, or finding pdf files downloaded from the Internet to my desktop and not knowing what they are nor how they got there. Or, like driving home from my doctor's office and forgetting what she said about medications and exercises for my bad back. And yet, when given a few clues, I can recall events of the more distant past with some clarity.

I've passed two psychological workups using standard tests for Alzheimer's in the last ten years – and scored even better on the second one. It is evident to me those tests are irrelevant in measuring memory damage from statin drugs.

What this suggests is memory files in my brain are still housing those memories – but the part of my brain that searches and retrieves the information is damaged, much like a computer hard drive going bad.

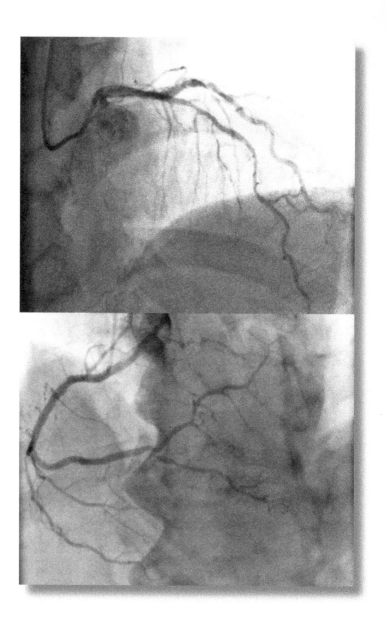

CHAPTER EIGHT

HOW COME DRUGS SEEM TO "CURE" ONLY SYMPTOMS?

At a press conference on July 2, 1992, Linus Pauling and Matthias Rath, MD presented their advances in vitamin research and the possible eradication of heart disease to the world. The pharmaceutical companies reacted immediately through the United States Food and Drug Administration (FDA). A nationwide campaign was started to prohibit all health claims in relation to vitamins and other natural substances. (https://tinyurl.com/p63k676)

Author's Disclosure: I received government pay checks for 24 years as a Navy officer (active and reserve) and in the decade of the 1970's (as chief environmental spokesman for the state of Maine). I started several businesses that did not survive long term. Yet I remain an unabashed advocate for capitalism. The profit motive is what made the United States prosper.

When it comes to our health, though, there is a cloud over the issue of decisions based on profits. In the past, the impact was thought to be felt mostly by those with "orphan diseases" (defined in the U.S. as illnesses with a prevalence of fewer than 200,000 individuals at any given time), which lacked research dollars mostly because there was no profit in it.

As I write this, however, new reports place us all at risk. Critical shortages have developed in drugs used in operating rooms as well as at local pharmacies. The situation is serious enough that some patients have died. The U.S. Food and Drug Administration now maintains a website, "Current Drug Shortages" (http://tinyurl.com/ycwg5lva). It also offers this site (https://tinyurl.com/yapgqos6), where you can subscribe so that you will be alerted if a drug you are taking is on the list.

Why is this happening? The Institute for Safe Medication Practices, the American Society for Health System Pharmacists (ASHP), the American Society of Clinical Oncology (ASCO), the American Society of Anesthesiologists (ASA) and the American Hospital Association (AHA) are studying the causes. In one of its papers, though, the Institute for Safe Medication Practices (https://tinyurl.com/y7kptoq4) has called for "More effective FDA oversight, a comprehensive early warning system, and patient safety **and outcomes placed ahead of anyone's profit margins** ..." (Emphasis mine)

Without profits, there would be no private sector pharmaceutical industry. But trouble arises when our traditional profit motive seems to guide decisions that run counter to the reality of our health care needs. I don't pretend to have a solution.

§

Have you noticed the money Big Pharma makes peddling cures for *symptoms?*

Note: The previous edition of this book was able to cite several Internet pages where information on pharmaceutical industry profits was widely available. Between 2012 and mid-2017, however, that information has become scarce. The best source as of this writing appears to be at Public Citizen (http://tinyurl.com/yd8yv6u6). Recently (Spring 2018) President Trump laid out a proposal to force drug prices lower.

Has it ever crossed your mind how much money those pharmaceutical companies stand to lose should a major disease actually be cured? Has any major disease been eradicated in your lifetime?

OK, in my long lifetime I have to concede, we pretty much wiped out polio, yellow fever, malaria, mumps and other childhood diseases. But most of those were long ago.

Granted, there's been progress, especially in the treatment of many forms of cancer. Lives have been extended. Some blood born cancers have been "cured," but the best most patients can say about their particular cancer is it is "in remission." Often, too, the cures have been based on radical surgeries, removing breasts, lungs, lymph glands and other affected organs. AIDS has been brought under control – by a trade off, to a lifetime of enslavement to expensive drugs.

I'm not saying there is one, but just "what if" someone has already come up with an honest solution for a disease that plagues us? Like cancer, or Alzheimer's, or diabetes? Perhaps a cure based on vitamins and minerals, and not on chemical drugs? Would Big Pharma, the AMA and AHA welcome it with open arms, knowing it would wipe out billions in profits?

Not if what they have appeared to do to promote their precious statin drugs and diminish the Pauling/Rath cure for coronary artery disease is any example.

§

Update. GlaxoSmithKline may have painted themselves into a corner on AIDS treatment. They succeeded in getting the daily dose of a maintenance drug for HIV, the precursor of AIDS, down to just one capsule, but the patent will expire in 2026. How to protect future profits? According to the Wall Street Journal (http://tinyurl.com/q9o5kag) in May 2015, Glaxo announced it was funding a joint venture with the University of North Carolina at Chapel Hill (UNC-CH) for research on a "shock and kill" approach to HIV. In other words, the only thing left to do was to find an actual cure.

Note: That report was in May 2015; as of this writing (Spring 2018), no breakthrough has been announced.

§

A big reason Big Pharma continues to diminish Dr. Rath, as they did Pauling, is his outspoken, unequivocal criticism. One example is his website, "What You Need to Know About the Fraudulent Nature of the Pharmaceutical Investment Business With Disease" (https://tinyurl.com/o7heeqw).

Linus Pauling had already experienced Big Pharma's backlash several years prior to his and Dr. Rath's heart cure announcement. As mentioned in Chapter 2, Pauling and a Dr. Cameron demonstrated that terminal cancer patients lived many years longer on massive doses of vitamin C alone than did others who received the recommended standard chemotherapy. You can read about their ordeal on the website "Natural Cancer Treatments" (http://tinyurl.com/yd86jdy3). There is also, "War Between Orthodox and Alternative Medicine" (https://tinyurl.com/ycyl2prf)

§

DOLLARS FOR DOCS – HOW INDUSTRY DOLLARS REACH YOUR DOCTORS

Some have calculated that the pharmaceutical industry spends twice the amount of money it spends on research in its efforts to manipulate public opinion. Besides the large sums they spend on media advertising campaigns, to convince you to "ask your doctor" about their latest, greatest patented miracle, Big Pharma spends millions directly to influence doctors.

An article in the September 7, 2011, Orlando Sentinel, headlined, "Florida doctors taking millions of dollars in Big Pharma money," (http://tinyurl.com/pspzavw) puts some local faces on the doctor influencing efforts of the pharmaceutical companies:

"Among those who were paid the most in Central Florida's five counties are Dr. Cxxxx Cxxxx, an Orlando researcher who received $918,938 from three drug companies; Jxxx Hxxx, a registered nurse in The Villages who was paid $111,295 by Eli Lilly; and Dr. Dxxxx Txxxxx, an endocrinologist at Florida Hospital Celebration Health who earned $67,509 from Lilly. (the newspaper reveals their full names, so I don't feel compelled to do so here – DHL)

"While some payments, such as those that support research, are necessary," the paper notes, "money paid to doctors to curry favor and encourage them to promote a company's medications crosses an ethical line, say industry watchdogs."

Beginning in 2013, federal law required all drug and medical-device companies to disclose the amount and purpose of payments they give providers. The revelations can be eye popping.

You can find out if, and how much, any doctor in the country has recently received in payments from drug and device companies. The site run by the Centers for Medicare & Medicaid Services (CMS) can be found at https://tinyurl.com/nypkyze.

ProPublica, the website for journalism in the public interest, has created a tool based on CMS data. In addition to what individual doctors are paid, their site discloses drug and device companies' gross payments to doctors as a group. Go to their site, "Dollars for Docs," at https://tinyurl.com/khe9n8y.

§

WHY ARE DRUGS SO EXPENSIVE?

Simple answer: because big pharma buys off politicians and regulators.

The following was part of an article that appeared in the Bradenton, FL, Times on Sunday, Nov 01, 2015 (http://tinyurl.com/y9bd5z9u):

"Pharmaceutical companies argue that they need to gouge in the U.S. (http://tinyurl.com/y7nqmzhe) in order to recover the enormous R&D costs of developing a new drug. There's no question that bringing a drug to market comes with enormous financial costs. Under this argument, the industry has been able to secure favorable conditions in the U.S. economy, including strict copyright laws with more generous provisions than the rest of the world.

"Thanks to legislation signed into law by former President George Bush, the industry also doesn't need to worry about negotiating with the federal government for drugs paid for by Medicare and Medicaid. That's against the law. Thanks to the Obama administration and aggressive lobbying on the industry's behalf during TPP negotiation, it will soon benefit from many of those conditions in other countries as well.

"However, instead of leveraging the industry to accept conditions that would help lower costs for American consumers, Big Pharma will simply continue to pad its bottom line and dole out campaign cash to the bipartisan politicians who do its bidding. In the last (2012) presidential election cycle, Big Pharma sprinkled more than $50 million (http://tinyurl.com/nnz2ccf) on candidates, plus another $30 million in the mid-terms. That's just donations and doesn't count the hundreds of millions spent on lobbying (2018 update: http://tinyurl.com/y9nmahrj) or the hundreds of millions they hand out to doctors (http://tinyurl.com/ycexseut) by way of inflated "speaking fees" to keep the prescription pads moving. That's a lot of money, but when you consider that prescription drug spending is nearly $350 billion (with a *b*) annually, it's a rather small cost of doing business.

"While the industry claims that its big nut is research and development, 9 out of the 10 top pharmaceutical companies spend more money on (sales and marketing) (http://tinyurl.com/gpkovzy) than R&D. With one of the highest profit margins of any industry on the planet—close to 30 percent—there's a lot left over. Much of that goes to eye-popping compensation (http://tinyurl.com/zoxqav2) for its CEOs."

§

If similar profits could be made peddling vitamins, do you suppose Big Pharma might be promoting vitamin therapy with equal gusto?

Your retirement fund or 401K may be reaping the benefits of pharmaceutical profits, but at what cost to your health?

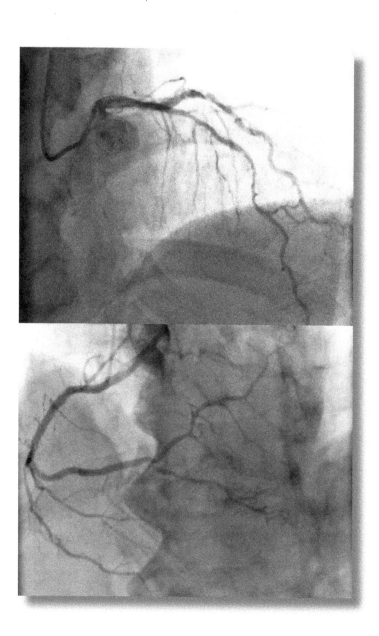

CHAPTER NINE

WHY WHAT YOU DON'T KNOW ABOUT STATIN DRUGS COULD, A) CRIPPLE YOU, OR B) WRECK YOUR BRAIN OR C) KILL YOU

"The Netherlands Radar TV Survey of Statin Side Effects:
"50,000 people were recently invited by e-mail to take part in an on-line survey by Radar Television in the Netherlands. "27,692 replied. Of these, 4738 (17.1%) were on Statins. Of the 4738, 27.1% reported side effects. They had a choice of: muscle pain, joint pain, digestion problems, loss of memory or other.

748 (39.8%) reported muscle pain
"592 (31.5%) reported joint pain
"301 (16.0%) reported digestion problems
"239 (12.7%) reported loss of memory
"420 reported other effects.
"To me this is perhaps as close as we have ever come to the true incidence of statin drugs side effects and it is very alarming. We know the usual breakdown of side effects - 40% cognitive, 40% muscle and 20 % all the rest but this is the first survey as to incidence that I feel I can believe."

—Duane Graveline, MD
(http://tinyurl.com/ya9serjk)

"LIPITOR is not for everyone. It is not for those with liver problems. And it is not for women who are nursing, pregnant or may become pregnant. If you take LIPITOR, tell your doctor if you feel any new muscle pain or weakness. This could be a sign of rare but serious muscle side effects. Tell your doctor about all medications you take. This may help avoid serious drug interactions. Your doctor should do blood tests to check your liver function before and during treatment and may adjust your dose. Common side effects are diarrhea, upset stomach, muscle and joint pain, and changes in some blood tests."
—the official Lipitor disclaimer (http://www.lipitor.com/)

What's a little "muscle and joint pain," compared to preventing heart attacks, you might wonder. The phrase is repeated so blithely at the end of TV commercials for statin drugs that it might go unnoticed. Unless, that is, you have experienced it first hand.

In my 17 years of taking statin drugs, the pattern kept repeating. After anywhere from six to eighteen months, I would develop a dull ache. For me, it was always in the same spot, just beneath the lowest rib on my right side. It would gradually increase from that dull ache to a stabbing pain. "It can't be the statin," my doctors would say, "but let's take you off of it and see what happens." After a few days off the drug, invariably my pain would go away.

As luck would have it, another newly patented synthetic statin drug would have recently come on the market – reflecting the constant need of the industry to stay a step ahead of patent expirations, when generic mimics of the original drug flood the market and drive profits down. My then-heart doctor would start me on this latest "miracle," and the pattern would be repeated.

Until, that is, we got to Lipitor. I thought I had finally found my simpatico statin. I was two-and-a half years into Lipitor, thinking all was fine. One night, talking with my cousin, a former nursing home employee, I said my hips had been aching a lot lately. Her immediate response was, "Are you taking Lipitor?"

At her urging, I went to see my new heart doctor a few days later. I asked him whether my aching hips could be related to the statin. "Let's find out," he said. "Stop taking it and let's see what happens."

What happened next shocked me. While the pain in my side subsided, I suddenly developed excruciating pain in the big muscles of both legs. It got so painful that one day when I went to a Home Depot store I had to grab a shopping carriage in the parking lot just to keep myself upright. At the back of the store the pain became so intense I did not know whether I was going to make it back to my car. I believe what I experienced was a form of statin drug withdrawal.

"It couldn't have been the Lipitor," my new heart doctor exclaimed. "Statins don't do that," said my family doctor. Oddly, though, my leg pains gradually subsided. They were completely gone six weeks after stopping Lipitor, and they have never come back.

2018 update: According to the New York Times, http://tinyurl.com/ofxy5za [13th paragraph)] Johns Hopkins researchers in 2010 found that this can happen in a small minority of patients. It occurs when statin drugs trigger a person's own antibodies to injure muscle tissue.

"This could be a sign of rare but serious muscle side effects," the TV statin spokesperson opines in that famous low-key monotone disclaimer we've all heard hundreds of times. Well, it turns out, those serious side effects have a name.

Rhabdomyolysis is the breakdown of muscle fibers resulting in the release of muscle fiber contents (myoglobin) into the bloodstream. Some of these are harmful to the kidneys and frequently result in kidney damage. Your doctor knows this, and now you know why he or she sends you twice yearly for blood tests if you are on a statin drug. They are monitoring the drug's effects on your kidneys. See https://tinyurl.com/y7mnwbeq

NOW, THE KICKER

The asterisk tells the true story.

In a moment of candor, Pfizer ran this print ad in 2009. In the very fine print (lower left), it admitted, "That means in a large clinical study, 3% of patients taking a sugar pill or placebo had a heart attack compared to 2% of patients taking Lipitor."

Let that sink in.

Big Pharma likes to confuse us with something called

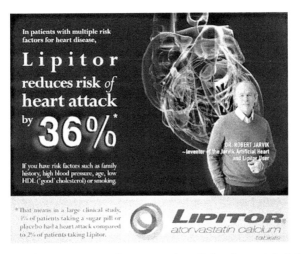

In patients with multiple risk factors for heart disease,

L i p i t o r
reduces risk *of*
heart attack
by **36%***

If you have risk factors such as family history, high blood pressure, age, low HDL ('good' cholesterol) or smoking.

DR. ROBERT JARVIK
—Inventor of the Jarvik Artificial Heart and Lipitor User

* That means in a large clinical study, 3% of patients taking a sugar pill or placebo had a heart attack compared to 2% of patients taking Lipitor.

LIPITOR
atorvastatin calcium
tablets

"relative risk," as opposed to actual or "absolute risk." There's an old saying, "Figures lie, and liars figure."

Here's how you make 36% out of what is actually a minimal difference (in reality, it was 1.1%). In the group that got Lipitor, 98.1% survived. In the placebo group, 97% survived. So you take the difference between the two numbers (1.1%) and divide it by the death rate (3%) of the placebo group, and voila! "Lipitor reduces risk of heart attack by 36%!"

For an illustrated discussion of the above, check out the YouTube video, "An Update on Demonization and Deception in Research on Saturated Fat," (http://tinyurl.com/gkv7cju) **by Professor David M. Diamond of the University of South Florida.** The discussion of statin drugs begins at the 34-minute mark. However, if you would like to view an eye opening discussion about how to truly lose weight, start the video from the beginning.

§

In Chapter Seven we discussed the important role cholesterol plays in your brain. It is vital to the formation of new synapses, the channels that connect individual cells and make it possible for you to think. I described the permanent damage to my own cognitive processes that I attribute to 17 years on statin drugs. We also learned from Dr. Graveline's book, *Statin Drugs Side Effects,* of a study that found "100% of patients placed on statins showed measurable decrease in cognitive function after six months, whereas 100% of placebo treated control patients showed measurable increase in cognitive function during the same time period."

Here is Dr. Graveline on the mechanism by which statins impair memory: "Statin Damage to the Mevalonate Pathway," (web link: https://tinyurl.com/yb376dwv)

§

In a little reported "drug safety announcement" (http://tinyurl.com/yaybv2x8) in February, 2012, the FDA grudgingly took note that statin drugs are related to memory loss. This event went unnoticed, even by some of us who are deeply concerned about this issue. The FDA now requires – buried deep in those tiny print data sheets included with every statin prescription (which most of us never read) – the following words:

Memory loss and confusion have been reported with statin use. These reported events were generally not serious and went away once the drug was no longer being taken.

WHAT YOU DON'T KNOW ABOUT STATIN DRUGS

That has not been my experience. And as AARP reported in an article, "*10 Drugs That May Cause Memory Loss*" (http://tinyurl.com/m6mdmah), Number 2 on their list is statin drugs: three out of four people using these drugs experienced adverse cognitive effects "probably or definitely related to" the drug. The researchers also found that "90 percent of the patients who stopped statin therapy reported improvements in cognition, sometimes within days."

In other words, ten percent (thousands, if not millions, of real people like me) experience memory loss that may be permanent or long lasting.

My wife and I recently drove from Florida to Missouri. I mapped the route in advance. Yet, when a friend asked for details after our trip, I could not tell him route numbers, states we passed through, nor exactly where we encountered the fierce winter storm through which I had driven. I'm glad the FDA considers this "generally not serious." What's a little memory loss, as long as Big Pharma's profits keep rolling in?

Do not fall for the drug industry's call to put ever more Americans on statin drugs. I was on them for 17 years (and off them since 2007). I can tell you, statins are a hazard no one should endure.

Now – as reported by maverick doctor Joseph Mercola, DO, in his web article, "Do You Take Any of These 11 Dangerous Statins or Cholesterol Drugs?" (http://tinyurl.com/2f9kg7d) – Big Pharma is after your kids:

"*In a bold attempt to increase profits before the patent (ran out in 2011), Pfizer … introduced a chewable kid-friendly*

*version of Lipitor." "…seeking to boost sales of the drug,
children have become the new target market, and the conventional medical establishment is more than happy to oblige."*

Next, meet Senior Research Scientist at MIT (Massachusetts
Institute of Technology), Stephanie Seneff, and her report, *"A
Recipe for Alzheimer's Disease"* (http://tinyurl.com/yc7x84jd),
in which she notes:

> *"Indeed, a population-based study showed that people
> who had **ever taken** (emphasis mine, DHL) statins had
> an increased risk to Alzheimer's disease … More alarm-
> ingly, people who used to take statins had a hazard ratio
> of 2.54 (over two and a half times the risk of Alzheimer's)
> compared to people who never took statins.*

> *"What I think is happening is that the doctor is taking
> the patient off the statin drug once memory problems
> are noted, suspecting that the statin may be causing the
> problem. But it may well be too late at that point to
> recover. In my own studies on patient-provided drug side
> effect reports, I found a statistically significant increase in
> the mention of words and phrases associated with memory
> problems (p=0.011) in the statin drug reports compared to
> age-matched reports on a variety of other drugs."*

Dr. Seneff explains further:

> *"Americans have been well trained over the past few
> decades to avoid dietary fat and cholesterol and to stay
> out of the sun. Their conscientious implementation of
> this misguided advice has led to an epidemic in obesity*

and heart disease, along with a host of other debilitating conditions like arthritis and Alzheimer's disease.

"Cholesterol is to animals as chlorophyll is to plants. Cholesterol, absent from plants, is what gives animals mobility and a nervous system. It is therefore not surprising that statin drug side effects mainly impact muscles and the nervous system.

"The heart, as a muscle, is not exempt from statin toxicity. This is why the incidence of heart failure has steadily risen in step with the widespread adoption of statin therapy, now displacing cardiovascular disease as the number one killer. "In this article I am going to take you on a whirlwind tour of the 60,000 foot view of my understanding of the principle causes of the current health crisis in America.

"My extensive research has caused me to hypothesize a remarkable feat that the human body can perform in the presence of sunlight, which is to extract sulfur from hydrogen sulfide in the air and convert it to sulfate, taking advantage of the sun's energy to catalyze the reaction.

"This process takes place in the skin upon sun exposure, and also in the endothelial cells lining blood vessels, and in the red blood cells, platelets, and mast cells in the blood. This feat is performed by a very interesting molecule called "endothelial nitric oxide synthase," a misnomer, since its main responsibility is to synthesize sulfate rather than nitric oxide.

"The sulfate so produced plays a huge role in cardiovascular health, both by preventing blood clots and by keeping pathogenic microbes (bacteria and viruses) at bay. But it also plays another role that is just as important, which is to give cholesterol (as well as vitamin D and other sterols) a free ride through the blood stream.

"Vitamin D3 (a highly touted nutrient) is synthesized in the skin from cholesterol (a highly demonized nutrient) and its chemical structure is almost identical to that of cholesterol. By attaching to cholesterol or vitamin D3, sulfate makes the molecule water soluble, and this means that it no longer has to travel packaged up inside an LDL particle. LDL, as you probably know, is the so-called "bad" cholesterol, which will cause doctors to prescribe statins if the level is too high.

"A great way to lower LDL levels is to get adequate sun exposure. It's not going to work to take a vitamin D supplement: you have to go outside and soak up the sun, because supplements are never sulfated and vitamin D is not cholesterol. Raw cow's milk is the only dietary source I know of that actually supplies sulfated vitamin D3, but even that is still not cholesterol sulfate.

"Because most Americans have inadequate cholesterol in their skin and grossly inadequate amounts of sun exposure, they suffer from a huge deficiency in cholesterol and sulfate supply to the tissues. Not surprisingly, most impacted are the muscles and nervous system.

"Because the heart muscle is indispensable, the body has developed a back-up strategy to give it special treatment, which is to synthesize cholesterol sulfate from LDL and homocysteine in the fatty deposits (plaque) that build up in arteries supplying the heart. The macrophages in the plaque extract cholesterol from damaged small dense LDL particles, and export it to HDL-A1. The platelets in the plaque will only accept cholesterol from HDL-A1, which they then convert to cholesterol sulfate.

"They obtain the sulfate through yet another process which requires energy and oxidizing agents, extracting the sulfur from homocysteine. With insufficient homocysteine, the sulfur will most likely be extracted from cartilage, which gets its strength from extensive disulfide bonds. This, in my view, is the main cause of arthritis – depletion of sulfur from the cartilage in the joints. So now you have both cardiovascular disease and arthritis as a consequence of a low-fat diet and aggressive sun avoidance.

"Statin drugs dramatically lower LDL levels by interfering with cholesterol synthesis, and this wreaks havoc on the liver, the main back-up supplier of cholesterol to the tissues when cholesterol intake and cholesterol sulfate production are down. With the American diet, the liver has another huge task, which is to convert fructose to fat.

"The fat cannot be stored or shipped (via LDL) if there is insufficient cholesterol. As a consequence, the liver abandons this task, and the fructose builds up in

the blood, causing extensive glycation damage to blood proteins. One of the impacted proteins is the apoB in LDL, which interferes with LDL's ability to deliver its goods to the tissues, including cholesterol, fats, vitamins A, D, E, and K, and antioxidants. So LDL levels fall sharply with statins, and so does the bioavailability of all these nutrients.

"Muscle cells come to the rescue, heroically, by extracting excess fructose from the blood and converting it to lactate, using anaerobic metabolism. They have to switch over to anaerobic metabolism anyway, because coenzyme Q10, another casualty of statin therapy, is in low supply. Coenzyme Q10 is crucial for aerobic metabolism.

"Lactate is a great fuel for the heart and liver, but the problem is that the muscle cells get wrecked in the process, due to massive overdoses of fructose, in the context of inadequate cholesterol, which would have offered some protection. This is a principle contributor to the excessive muscle pain and weakness associated with statins. Eventually, the muscles can't do it anymore, and you're now on the verge towards heart failure.

"People on long-term statin therapy start to notice that their hair is receding faster, they're developing cataracts, they can't hear as well as they used to, they keep forgetting things, they can't open the pickle jar any more, and perhaps they'll need rotator cuff surgery soon, as their shoulders are so sore. They think it's just because they're growing old, but these are all side effects that my research, together *with my students at MIT, has uncovered, by comparing statin drug side effects with side effects associated with other drugs in age-matched reviews.*

"Even more alarming are the rare but debilitating and even life-threatening side effects we've detected, such as ALS and Parkinson's disease, heart and liver failure, neuropathy and severe muscle damage. A 17-year study on the elderly confirmed what I already suspected: low serum cholesterol is associated with increased frailty, accelerated mental decline, and early death (Ref 1).

"Statins are not the answer for anyone seeking to avoid cardiovascular disease. The answer, instead, is to modify the diet to include foods that are rich in cholesterol and saturated fat, to avoid empty carbohydrates, especially high fructose corn syrup, to eat foods that are good sources of sulfur, and, most especially, to spend plenty of time outdoors in the sun.

(The above is reprinted by permission of Dr. Seneff, with thanks to SpaceDoc.com – DHL)

§

Lastly, here is Dr. Mercola's interview (http://tinyurl.com/ykckdww) with the founder of THINCS, The International Network of Cholesterol Skeptics (www.thincs.org) Uffe Ravnskov, MD, PhD.

Dr. Mercola: "Specifically, what are your views on statins?"

"Their benefit is trivial, and has been seen only in male patients who already have heart disease.

"Worse is that their many adverse effects are ignored or cleverly belittled by the trial directors. Independent researchers have found many more and in much higher numbers. If they are true it means that today millions of previously healthy people probably consider their weak and painful muscles, their bad memory, their sexual failure, and their cancer to be a consequence of increasing age, and so do their doctors.

"The risk of cancer is most alarming. Both animal experiments, epidemiological studies and several of the statin trials have shown that low cholesterol predisposes to cancer.

"The widespread use of statin treatment probably explains why the decrease of the smoking habit that has been going on in many countries hasn't been followed by a decrease of cancer mortality. We should have seen a decrease because smoking predispose not only to bronchial cancer, but to all kinds of cancer."

FINAL THOUGHTS ON THIS CHAPTER

If a doctor has you on a statin drug, but has not told you to take the supplement Coenzyme Q10 (or CoQ10), he or she might be setting you up for memory issues, or even premature death, either from a heart attack or other organ failure. CoQ10 is a key factor in energy transfer inside your body's individual living cells.

Statin drugs block cholesterol production through something called the "mevalonate pathway." Unfortunately, cholesterol is not the only traveler along this pathway. It shares the space with CoQ10, among other things.

So, when statins block this pathway, they also hinder the body's uptake of CoQ10. Not only that, our bodies' ability to synthesize CoQ10 begins decreasing after age 21. For most of us over age 50, the only way to maintain an adequate level of CoQ10 is through over-the-counter supplements. Few of us bother, making the potential impact from the blocking function of statin drugs all that much worse.

Ironically, doctors put us on statins to protect our heart arteries. Yet, the heart is usually the first organ to be affected by low levels of CoQ10. That's because the heart requires the most energy of any bodily organ to keep working. What appears to be cardio- myopathy or congestive heart failure might actually be the result of too little CoQ10. But you won't see CoQ10 deficiency on a death certificate.

FURTHER READING

Following is a suggested reading list taken from the website for The International Network of Cholesterol Skeptics (THINCS) (http://www.thincs.org/news.htm)

John von Radowitz, (The Independent): 85% of new drugs 'offer few benefits' (http://tinyurl.com/2c8atl8)

Christopher Hudson (Telegraph), Wonder drug that stole my memory (http://tinyurl.com/ybwsdomt). Statins have been hailed as a miracle cure for cholesterol, but little is known about their side effects. Read also the comments that follow the article, but beware, they are scary.

Melinda Wenner Moyer (Scientific American), It's Not Dementia, It's Your Heart Medication: Cholesterol Drugs and Memory. Why cholesterol drugs might affect memory. (http://tinyurl.com/zjh2gsj)

Tom Naughton, Big Fat Fiasco: how the misguided fear of saturated fat created a nation of obese diabetics (http://tinyurl.com/22q7z86). A humourous speech with a serious content. Five parts, on Youtube

Uffe Ravnskov, Ignore the Awkward! How the Cholesterol Myths are Kept Alive (http://tinyurl.com/y9ntzskw). A book.about how prominent scientists have turned white into black by ignoring all conflicting observations; by twisting and exaggerating trivial findings; by citing studies with opposing results in a way to make them look supportive; and by ignoring or scorning the work of critical scientists. Includes a short and simplified version of his previous book

Denise Minger, The China Study: Fact or Fallacy (http://tinyurl.com/y8p77w3d). Is the book by that title, authored by Colin Campbell, really "one of the most important books about nutrition ever written", as stated on the cover by Dean Ornish? Or is it, rather, one of the most misleading? Read Minger's review.

David H. Freeman, Lies, Damned Lies and Medical Science (http://tinyurl.com/mrqpvgs). The Atlantic Nov. 2010

PublicCitizen, Dec 16, 2010: Rapidly Increasing Criminal and Civil Monetary Penalties Against the Pharmaceutical Industry: 1991 to 2010 (http://tinyurl.com/ycbjkgpo)

Malcolm Kendrick, The Cholesterol Myth exposed (http://tinyurl.com/y84uvf9u). A short Youtube presentation

Lipitor Paradox, A funny but also sad YouTube movie (http://tinyurl.com/q5n3ony) in support of Kendrick's findings.

Emily Deans, Low Cholesterol and Suicide (http://tinyurl.com/yam8z9fd).

Dwight D Lundell, The Statin Scam (http://tinyurl.com/y9j4zf8m). A view from an experienced thoracic surgeon.

Stephanie Seneff, How Statins Really Work Explains Why They Don't Really Work (http://tinyurl.com/6zdjp9d).

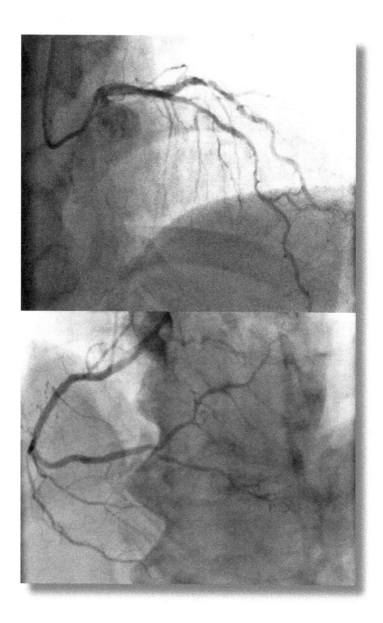

CHAPTER TEN

WOMEN AND STATIN DRUGS

I am obviously no expert, just a much concerned layman. My focus in this book has not been on gender. But I have received many inquiries about benefits or disadvantages of statin drugs for women. The following represent some of the news items I have gathered about women and statins over the last several years.

§

"To date, no large trial of women statin users who already have cardiovascular disease has been shown to increase life expectancy by one day. More importantly, the use of statins in women at lower risk has not increased life expectancy nor prevented heart attacks and stroke.

"It raises the question whether women should be prescribed statins at all. I believe that the answer is no. Statins fail to provide any overall health benefit in women.

"The more recent heart protection study was hailed as a success for men and women, but despite the hype there was no effect on mortality in women."

–The Great Cholesterol Con by Malcolm Kendrick
(https://tinyurl.com/y8zsssnq); John Blake Publishing

§

"In a smaller group of women — those who already have heart disease — the data suggests that statins can reduce heart-related deaths. But as Dr. Beatrice Golomb, a professor of medicine at the University of California, San Diego, says, they don't reduce deaths overall. 'Any reduction in death from heart disease seen in the data has been completely offset by deaths from other causes,' she says. Which raises the question: If statins do not help prolong women's lives, why are so many women taking them?"

–Time Magazine, March 29, 2010
(http://tinyurl.com/nn5bu94)

§

"For women with heart disease, using statin drugs reduces the chance they'll have a heart attack. But for some women—those who only have elevated LDL (or 'bad' cholesterol levels) with a very low risk for cardiovascular disease—the benefit of statins should be weighed against the potential harm from taking them."

– Consumer Reports, June 2010
(http://tinyurl.com/nkcrw7g)

§

"Women who take statins for more than a decade face double the risk of contracting the most common type of breast cancer."

"The latest findings identified invasive ductal carcinoma (IDC) which starts in the ducts of the breast before spreading inwards. It accounts for around seven out of ten breast cancer cases."

"The experts at the Fred Hutchinson Cancer Research Centre in Seattle, US, also found the chances of getting invasive lobular carcinoma, which accounts for ten to 15 per cent of breast cancers, went up almost 2.5 times in some women on statins long-term."

"The researchers said one explanation may be that statins affect hormone regulation in the body, especially as the study found women on the drugs were significantly more likely to suffer cancers driven by the hormone estrogen."

–The above four paragraphs excerpted
from U.K. Daily Mail Online, July 19, 2013
and written by Pat Hagan (http://tinyurl.com/ljc8866)

§

"Based on unabated rates of cardiovascular disease despite a generation of statin users, and studies that demonstrate that patients presenting to the hospital with heart attacks don't have elevated total cholesterol, but they do have (66 percent of the time) metabolic syndrome, or a constellation of findings such as obesity, high triglycerides, low HDL, and insulin resistance. This phenomenon is driven by sugar and trans fat, not dietary, naturally-occurring saturated fat, and not by a lack of statins, but,

perhaps, is exacerbated by the statins themselves, and particularly, in women."

> – Kelly Brogan, MD, in Huffpost Blog 11/20/2013
> (http://tinyurl.com/muqo3ju)

§

"'The data are underwhelming, to say the least,' said Dr. Barbara Roberts, author of 'The Truth About Statins: Risks and Alternatives to Cholesterol-Lowering Drugs' and an associate professor of medicine at Brown University. 'Women who are healthy derive no benefit from statins, and even those women who have established heart disease derive only half the benefit men do.'

"Dr. C. Noel Bairey Merz, director of the Barbra Streisand Women's Heart Center at the Cedars-Sinai Heart Institute in Los Angeles, disagreed. 'We haven't shown that we can prevent deaths, because we just haven't enrolled enough women, and that's a crime,' she said. 'But the absence of data is not the same as negative data.'

"In the meantime, she said, 'we can either sit on our hands or use our best judgment to make an educated guess, and can decide to treat.' **(Dr. Bairey Merz has had financial relationships with drug companies, including Abbott Vascular, Bristol-Myers Squibb and Gilead.)**" (Bold Italics mine –DHL)

> – The New York Times blog, May 5, 2014
> (http://tinyurl.com/ofxy5za)

§

"If you are a post-menopausal women (sic) with high cholesterol, your doctor will almost certainly recommend cholesterol lowering medication or statins. And it just might kill you. A new study in the Archives of Internal Medicine found that statins increase the risk of getting diabetes by 71 percent in post-menopausal women.

"Since diabetes is a major cause of heart disease, this study calls into question current recommendations and guidelines from most professional medical associations and physicians. The recommendation for women to take statins to prevent heart attacks (called primary prevention) may do more harm than good."

– Dr. Mark Hyman, MD, October 18, 2014
(http://tinyurl.com/mh2dxu4)

§

"Statins are often prescribed for older women with high levels of blood cholesterol, yet the effects of the drug have not been as well-studied in this group as in others. Now, a new study from Australia finds that older women taking statins to lower cholesterol may have a significantly higher risk of developing diabetes."

– Catharine Paddock PhD, Medical News Today,
March 16, 2017 (https://tinyurl.com/y8g7dnaq)

§

"An analysis of data from the Systolic Blood Pressure Intervention Trial (SPRINT) shows that people over 65 or 70 do not appear to benefit from statin-type cholesterol-lowering medicine (JAMA Internal Medicine, online, Jan. 22, 2018). There were

over 9,000 men and women recruited for the SPRINT trial. They did not have cardiovascular disease at the start of the study but they all had hypertension. Some of these patients were taking statins when they entered the study. Even though these older adults were at relatively high risk for cardiovascular events, statins did not protect them."

"This new research analysis published in JAMA Internal Medicine will come as a shock to many physicians. Those health professionals who relied upon the AHA and ACC guidelines will likely be annoyed by this report. After all, experts in the cardiology community are supposed to make decisions and recommendations based on the scientific evidence. They have been advocating statins to prevent a first heart attack (primary prevention) for years."

–Joe Graedon, The People's Pharmacy online
(https://tinyurl.com/yc2wg2jg), January 25, 2018

CHAPTER ELEVEN

IF YOUR DOCTOR SAYS "DON'T TRY THIS," FIND ANOTHER DOCTOR

"Any physician, or panel of hospital-based physicians, claiming that vitamin C is experimental, unapproved, and/or posing unwarranted risks to the health of the patient, is really only demonstrating a complete and total ignorance or denial of the scientific literature. A serious question as to what the real motivations might be in the withholding of such a therapy then arises..... ignorance of medical fact is ultimately no sound defence for a doctor withholding valid treatment, especially when that information can be easily accessed."

—Thomas E. Levy, M.D., J.D.
http://tinyurl.com/yb9dm6s6

My first cardiologist treated me from age 48 to 63. He implanted those three hated stents in my heart in September, 2003. In January 2004 he issued the letter of "permanent limitation" you see displayed right after the Introduction of this book. A year later, his group of physicians elected to no longer accept the insurance plan I had at that time. Disappointed, I was left with no choice but to find a new heart doctor, so I don't know how the first one might have reacted to my vitamin C regimen. I have not seen him since.

I was with my next cardiologist for six years, until we relocated from Winter Park, FL, to Bradenton on the Gulf Coast. When I eventually developed serious side effects from the Lipitor – as I'd had with all the other available statins – my Winter Park doctor was stumped. He actually said, "There's nothing more I can do for you." But when I brought him the results of my Internet research – the Pauling/Rath patented cure for heart disease – he was skeptical yet open minded. He agreed to work with me to monitor my condition. This included checkups, ordering fasting blood tests, and occasional stress tests. I had to agree to continue taking four other prescription medications plus low-dose aspirin. Eventually, I stopped taking all prescription medications and the aspirin.

My family doctor in Winter Park, too, was supportive. I think he was skeptical, but he never said so to my face. He, too, monitored my condition, and he was dually impressed with the results of my July 2011 angiography. He had to agree, upon viewing those photos of my artery x-rays as shown throughout this book, and reading the cardiac interventionist's report, my coronary artery disease was gone.

Since moving to Bradenton I have again found a family doctor and a heart specialist willing to "treat" me by simply monitoring my health. As noted in the new Chapter 2 of this book, I broke Linus Pauling's cardinal rule: "Never miss a day." At the behest of the gastroenterologist I was seeing at the time, and for sixteen months I took no Vitamin C. As you've seen in that chapter, I paid a high price.

As of this 2018 update, I am age 76 and have been back on Vitamin C for more than a year. My health is not what it was prior to my two additional stents in December of 2015, but I still get around pretty well.

As this book was going to print (June 2018), it was discovered I have a blocked and collapsed middle lobe of my right lung. Thankfully, despite two biopsies, no cancer has been found. In case future surgery is needed, though, my pulmonologist suggested I see my heart doctor for a preparatory stress test. My heart doctor was amazed. He commented that reading my results was "extremely easy." Thank you, Linus Pauling and Matthias Rath!

My advice to you is this. There are a growing number of cardiologists and family doctors who have heard about the Pauling/Rath Protocol, and an increasing number who are open minded enough to work with patients who want to try it. How far that openness extends may depend, in part, on how well your body has responded to his or her preferred treatment with statin drugs. Remember, I had actually run out of statin options.

The point is, if, having read this book and after conducting your own additional research, you want to pursue the Pauling/

Rath protocol, there are doctors out there who will work with you. Don't be afraid to interview several until you find the right fit. And, above all, don't go it alone. Remember the old adage; he who treats himself has a fool for a doctor.

Start by discussing this with your current doctor(s). If you are met with resistance, start interviewing replacements.

2018 Update: Another miracle of vitamin C reported by Dr. Levy (see his quote leading off this chapter): *"Vitamin C and Sepsis, The genie is now out of the bottle"* (https://tinyurl.com/ycoa8j3r)

Admittedly, the above is not the focus of this book. But I've known two women stricken by sepsis in the past year. One died. The other was hospitalized many weeks and finally pulled through. If you or a family member sometime faces this, the most common killer of hospitalized patients, remember Dr. Levy's article. It might save a life.

MY ACTUAL DAILY INTAKE
AND WHY I TAKE ALL THOSE PILLS

It probably helped that I grew up in a home where my mother was an ardent reader of Prevention Magazine. She took several vitamins, and she started me on a children's multi-vitamin at an early age. I don't think she obsessed about them, but that magazine had lots of articles about the benefits of vitamins for this or that human condition. Let's just say my childhood experience made me open minded on the subject of vitamins and minerals.

I was in my forties, though, before I took much more than an adult one-a-day type of multi-vitamin. At some point, I began on my own – but always with my doctors' awareness – to expand into what some might consider more naturopathic uses of vitamins and minerals to promote wellness and prevent illness.

2018 Update: Always check for safe limits of any supplement you consider taking, and search online for any possible adverse effects. I take some comfort, however, in these annual reports from the U.S. National Poison Data System, published in the journal Clinical Toxicology, as reported by the *Orthomolecular. org* News Service: *"No Deaths from Vitamins. None."* (https:// tinyurl.com/y7gap6ng) and *"No Deaths from Supplements. No Deaths from Minerals or Amino Acids. No Deaths from Homeopathics or Herbs."* (https://tinyurl.com/ycg6j3ql).

Compare the above with this 2006 article: *Drug Errors Send 700,000 to ER Every Year* (http://tinyurl.com/o4bts72).

At any rate, let's look at what's on my supplement menu for today … and why.

HEART

Baby Aspirin (81 mg), because of the two new stents I received in 2015, my current heart doctor insisted I take this indefinitely. We argued about it, and he finally agreed I could take one every three days – the stuff stays in your blood stream that long anyway. That was our compromise if I wanted to keep him as my doctor, and I do. I still must put up with some bruising (mostly on my arms), but nothing like the amount I had with the daily aspirin regimen.

Vitamin C, 6,000 mg (6 grams) daily, divided in three equal doses. This is my maintenance dosage; for the first couple months I took 10,000 mg. (10 grams). See Chapter Four for details.

Note: See the **2018 Update** section of Chapter One for my recent (failed) attempt to boost my intake to 15 grams. As I write this I am again experimenting to find my body's upper tolerance level.

L-Lyzine, 3,000 mg daily, divided in three equal doses (using 500 mg capsules), to cleanse Lp(a) plaques from heart arteries. See Chapters One and Four for details.

L-Proline, 1,000 mg, (using one 500 mg capsule morning and night), also to prevent Lp(a) build up. See Chapters One and Four for details.

L-Arginine, 500 mg, one tablet daily in the AM for heart health. Recommended by Linus Pauling. See Chapters One and Four for details.

Fish Oil, morning and night, for its Omega-3 Fatty Acids which support heart health and also reduce blood clotting. There is an expensive prescription alternative (with a little synthetic tweaking, I am told), but Consumer Labs deems it a prescription most folks don't need (https://tinyurl.com/y9b6m83c).

CoQ10, 100 mg, three times daily. If you are still on statin drugs, this is a MUST. I continue to take it to strengthen heart muscle and to counter the damage to heart and brain cells done over the 17 years I was on statin drugs.

BRAIN/NERVOUS SYSTEM

My greatest concern regarding my years on statin drugs has more to do with my head than my heart. If you have read Chapter Nine, you know about my memory issues. If you have not read the Duane Graveline, MD, book *Lipitor, Thief of Memory*, or visited his website, www.SpaceDoc.com, I hope you will do so without delay. That goes double if you are taking any form of statins.

Bacopa Extract, 500 mg morning and night. Bacopa is important in traditional Ayurvedic medicine. It has been used, particularly in India, for several thousand years. Recent studies have indicated it may aid memory and promote a sense of well-being. Quoting WebMD, "(Bacopa monnieri) might increase certain brain chemicals that are involved in thinking, learning, and memory."

As for myself, I do think it is helping. There was no "aha!" moment, but there's been a gradual release from the tension of trying to come up with the right word in conversation. I guess you could say I feel more confident, more relaxed, and I seem to be able to remember little things better. Like short shopping lists, or placing more names with faces of actors on TV shows or movies. Some days are better than others, but over all I believe it has helped.

CoQ10, (see HEART section, above). Statin drugs deprive the brain and other organs of this needed substance. Quoting Wikipedia, "This oil-soluble, vitamin-like substance is present in most eukaryotic cells, primarily in the mitochondria. It is a component of the electron transport chain and participates in aerobic cellular respiration, generating energy in the form of ATP. *Ninety-five percent of the human body's energy is generated this way.* Therefore, those organs with the highest energy requirements—such as the heart, liver and kidney —have the highest CoQ10 concentrations." (Emphasis mine –DHL)

PQQ (Pyrroloquinoline Quinone) 20 mg, a potent anti-oxidant, once daily in AM to improve brain health, added in 2014.

Phosphatidylserine, 100 mg three times daily. In May of 2003, the FDA gave it "qualified health claim" status, saying Phosphatidylserine "may reduce the risk of dementia and cognitive dysfunction in the elderly."

Vitamin B12, 1,000 mcg, once daily in the AM, to promote homocysteine for health of nervous system.

Cinnamon, 1000 mg capsule, two in AM and two in PM, recommended in 2014 by my osteopathic physician to help keep blood pressure in check without drugs. As I update this section, in 2018, there is new debate about what constitutes acceptable blood pressure in the elderly (I turned 76 at the end of January). While my systolic pressure runs just under or over 140 – formerly considered reasonable for my age – there is now a push to get everyone's pressure down to 100. Might this be the hand of Big Pharma looking to increase its bottom line, as was done with statin drugs? Hard to know for sure.

STOMACH

Antacid. Omeprazole 20 mg (generic for Prilosec 20 mg), prescribed by my gastroenterologist to control Gastro-Intestinal Distress (GURD). The kicker is there is a small probability that this and all other proton pump inhibitors might contribute to the development of heart disease. Too, because a proton pump inhibitor may have caused my (temporary) microscopic colitis, I am in an ongoing debate with my current gastroenterologist, who wants me to take a PPI indefinitely. I also use over-the-counter antacid tablets as needed.

Folic Acid, 800 mcg, once daily, to boost pancreatic health/insulin production.

Probiotic Supplement, one capsule daily in the AM. Recommended by a nutritionist to keep "good" bacteria flourishing in my gut. I purchase the Schiff Digestive Advantage brand for its promise to survive passage through stomach acids and deliver a greater quantity of healthy bacteria to colonize the small intestine.

Vitamin B6, 50 mg, one tablet daily in the AM., to boost pancreatic health/insulin production Based on "dangerously high" blood levels of B6 in 2015, my family doctor urged me to discontinue it. I do listen to medical advice, some of the time.

JOINT HEALTH

Glucosamine/Chondroitin, 1500 mg/1200 mg, respectively; one tablet in AM and one at night. I have been taking this for several years and it seems to be working. At age 76, I can still deep knee bend, stand and walk without pain.

BONE HEALTH

Magnesium w/Chelated Zinc, 400 mg/15 mg, one tablet morning and night.

MUSCLE HEALTH

Potassium Gluconate, 99 mg, one tablet daily in AM to prevent muscle cramping. I began taking this to ward off the effects of statin drugs, and have continued it to preserve muscle tone.

VISION

Lutein plus Zeaxanthin Isomers, 20 mg/2 mg, one capsule every morning, on the recommendation of my ophthalmologist.

Vision Formula vitamin capsule (eQuate Brand from Walmart), 1 tablet every morning, and so far no cataracts – or at least not developed enough to warrant surgery.

Astaxanthin, 4 mg, every morning (added in 2014) is said to have many health benefits. It's been linked to healthier skin, endurance, heart health, and joint pain.

SENIOR HEALTH

"Mature Adult Multi-Vitamin," (Centrum Silver, recommended as best by ConsumerLab.com) one tablet daily in the morning. Linus Pauling recommended taking an adult multi-vitamin. I take it in addition to my other vitamins and supplements because it might fill in items I would not get otherwise. Remember that report from earlier, that on average there is one admission per year to American emergency rooms for anything vitamin related, but 700,000 Americans each year go to the ER for emergencies related to prescription medications.

Vitamin B50 Complex, once daily in the AM. This supplement contains 50% or more of the FDA recommended daily allowance of all the B vitamins. Remember, the "daily allowance" is FDA's best guess at the *minimum* amount of a particular vitamin or supplement our bodies need. That is how they concluded we need only 60 mg of vitamin C each day, versus the 6,000 mg or more in the Pauling/Rath protocol. I take this complex to complement my other sources of the B vitamins. Note: I had been taking B150, but blood work in early 2015 indicated my blood levels of B vitamins were getting too high.

ANTI-AGING

Resveratrol, 200 mg, one capsule daily at noon. This ingredient found in red wine was touted a few years ago by Barbara Walters, Dr. Oz and others because in laboratories it extended the lives of mice and lesser life forms. Perhaps it can do the same for humans. Time will tell (wry wit intended).

[See the discussion in Appendix B, regarding attempts by Big Pharma to corner this market, too.]

ALLERGIES

I took allergy shots for more than seven years but finished them in September of 2017. My allergies included most grasses, dust, mold, cats, etc. And then there's something those in my state call "Florida crud." My allergist now says I have late onset asthma (?!), but when I visit northern states it seems to diminish. He has me on two inhalers – Flovent HFA morning and night, and ProAir HFA as needed; they seem to help a bit.

ANTIOXIDENT

Selenium, 200 mcg, one tablet daily in the AM. Of course, Vitamin C and some of the other supplements I am taking serve secondarily as antioxidants, too.

Vitamin E, 400 iu, once daily in the AM. It has also been demonstrated to support cardio, prostate and overall health. If you have heard that this vitamin is "controversial," visit this Mayo Clinic website: https://tinyurl.com/y97cnhw3

IMMUNE SYSTEM

Vitamin D3, 400 IU, one tablet daily in the AM, supports the immune system and overall health. Of course, doctors will tell you, vitamin D is also important for bone health in the young and the old. Our bodies actually make vitamin D when exposed to the sun. Some of us, myself included, avoid the sun because of repeated bouts with skin cancer; so I avoid the sun (in Florida!) and rely on supplements. My ears, nose and parts of my face have had to have plastic surgery after skin cancer removal; the scars on my back from skin cancer removal (most recently, a malignant melanoma) would make you think I'd been in a knife fight.

PROSTATE HEALTH

Bee Pollen, 550 mg, one capsule morning and night. Twenty or more years ago, I read about Swedish research indicating that Bee Pollen and Zinc together delay or prevent enlargement of the male prostate gland. I have been taking them ever since. Blood tests to date indicate no signs of prostate cancer. Is my urine flow that of a young man? Uh, no. Golden flow is not a part of the Golden Years for us guys. Booklet: Prostate Disorders and Natural Medicine, by Rita Elkins (http://tinyurl. com/q2o5dnc).

Zinc, 50 mg, one tablet in the AM (see above).

Saw Palmetto, 540 mg, two capsules morning and night.

That's the sum of stuff I take on a daily basis. Whether and how much those other than the BIG FOUR (Vitamin C, L-Lyzine, L-Proline and L-Arginine) had any role in reversing my coronary artery disease is hard to say. Remember, this is the collection of vitamins and supplements I have chosen for myself. Many of them I have taken for years (before and subsequent to my coronary artery disease). I am not recommending them, and I am not a medical doctor. Every one of us is a unique individual, with unique needs. You and your doctor should decide what is best for you.

2018 Update: Recently, there were reports that some in-house vitamin brands from Walmart, Walgreens, CVS and other retailers failed to contain what was claimed on their labels. That caused me to subscribe to a website I highly recommend for you, too. *Consumer Lab* purchases supplement products on the open market and has them tested for quality by third party laboratories. You can learn more about them by going to http://tinyurl.com/r2gjy. Before purchasing any new over-the-counter supplement, I first check to see whether there is a Consumer Lab test result for that product (requires an inexpensive annual membership).

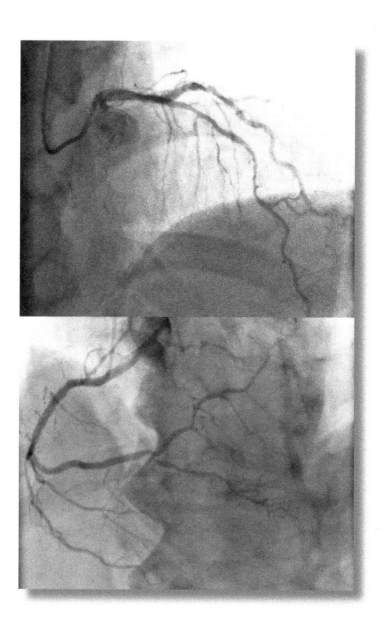

WILL YOU LET THE U.S. GOVERNMENT TAKE AWAY YOUR VITAMINS AND SUPPLEMENTS?

Orthomolecular Medicine News Service, January 5, 2017
(https://tinyurl.com/ycg6j3ql)
"No Deaths from Supplements. No Deaths from Minerals or Amino Acids. No Deaths from Homeopathics or Herbs."
by Andrew W. Saul, Editor

> *"Not only are there no deaths from vitamins, there are also **zero deaths from any supplement**. The most recent (2015) information collected by the U.S. National Poison Data System, and published in the journal Clinical Toxicology (1), shows **no deaths whatsoever** from dietary supplements.*
>
> *"No deaths from minerals*
>
> *"There were zero deaths from any dietary mineral supplement. This means there were no fatalities from calcium, magnesium, chromium, zinc, colloidal silver, selenium, iron,*

or multimineral supplements. Reported in the "Electrolyte and Mineral" category was a fatality from the medical use of "Sodium and sodium salts" and another fatality from non-supplemental iron, which was clearly and specifically excluded from the supplement category.

"No deaths from any other nutritional supplement

"Additionally, there were zero deaths from any amino acid or herbal product. This means no deaths at all from blue cohosh, echinacea, ginkgo biloba, ginseng, kava kava, St. John's wort, valerian, yohimbe, Asian medicines, ayurvedic medicines, or any other botanical. There were zero deaths from creatine, blue-green algae, glucosamine, chondroitin, or melatonin. There were zero deaths from any homeopathic remedy.

"But when in doubt, blame a supplement. Any supplement.

"There actually was one fatality alleged from some 'Unknown Dietary Supplement or Homeopathic Agent.' This is hearsay at best, and scaremongering at worst. How can an accusation be based on the unknown? Claiming causation without even knowing what substance or ingredient to accuse is baseless.

"The truth: no man, woman or child died from any nutritional supplement. Period.

*"If nutritional supplements are allegedly so 'dangerous,' as the FDA, the news media, and even some physicians still claim, then **where are the bodies**?"*

In Chapter Four we discussed how Big Pharma, together with the AMA and FDA, almost drove all naturopaths out of the medical practice. Thanks to organizations like Prevention, and later the advent of the Internet, vitamin and mineral producers and practitioners have survived and rebounded. And yet, American emergency rooms only see, on average, *one patient per year* with an adverse reaction to vitamins and minerals. They see an average 700,000 per year due to pharmaceutical side effects and/or overdoses (1 million per year as of 2017: http://tinyurl.com/pwwhgvo).

None of that can explain this.

Just as I was putting the finishing touches on (the first edition of) this book, I was made aware of efforts to thwart our access to these non-prescription products. The back story is pretty ugly. Long held patents are running out on the block buster cash cows of Big Pharma, and profits stand to plummet. If they can create synthetic (and thereby patentable) versions of the stuff we get now over the counter – and at the same time drive prices of the natural versions out of sight, their good times can continue . . . at our expense.

One example is resveratrol. This ingredient found in red wine was touted a few years ago by Barbara Walters, Dr. Oz and others because it may have anti-aging properties. One U.S. manufacturer, a small company called Sirtris, was purchased for $720 million in 2008 by GlaxoSmithKline. According to an article that appeared in the New York Times (http://tinyurl.com/4os6qmz), the pharmaceutical giant cancelled clinical trials. Among reasons the Times pointed to was this "In addition, from a commercial point of view, resveratrol is a natural substance and not patentable." GSM bought Sirtis, the Times opined, because its research facilities might be able to create a synthetic (and thereby patentable) version of resveratrol.

Direct acquisition of all the vitamin and supplement manufacturers, though, would cost Big Pharma a bundle – not to mention the bad publicity. But suppose, with a little help from their friends in Congress, and their lackeys in the U.S. Food & Drug Administration, they might drive prices of vitamins and supplements sky high? The little manufacturers would fall by the wayside. Big Pharma could pick up the slack, charging prescription prices or, even better, gaining prescription status for synthetic knock offs of the real things.

Their most blatant attempt to date was the "Dietary Supplement Labeling Act of 2011" (S. 1310), sponsored by Senator Richard Durbin (D-IL) (https://tinyurl.com/yctn7bzj), and reintroduced in 2013 (https://tinyurl.com/ya92kdcl)

Writer and Critical Care Nurse Byron J. Richards, chronicled the efforts of Durbin and the FDA:

- FDA Propaganda Attempts to Destroy the Dietary Supplement Industry, 8-23-11 (http://tinyurl.com/p7q7cl7)
- The FDA's Scheme to Reclassify Nutrients as Drugs, 8-3-11 (http://tinyurl.com/3z4q9cd)
- Senator Durbin and the FDA Viciously Attack Dietary Supplements, 7-26-11 (http://tinyurl.com/3zmawek)

As recently as 2015 attacks on dietary supplements were still ongoing: https://tinyurl.com/ybukmx6e.

2018 Update. Durbin's legislation failed to be approved by the U.S. Senate. However, the FDA is not without a presence in regulation of the Dietary Supplement industry. See its "Dietary Supplements Guidance Documents & Regulatory Information" (https://tinyurl.com/y9q4v2a5).

Bottom line: If you like your supplements and want to keep them, *stay vigilant.*

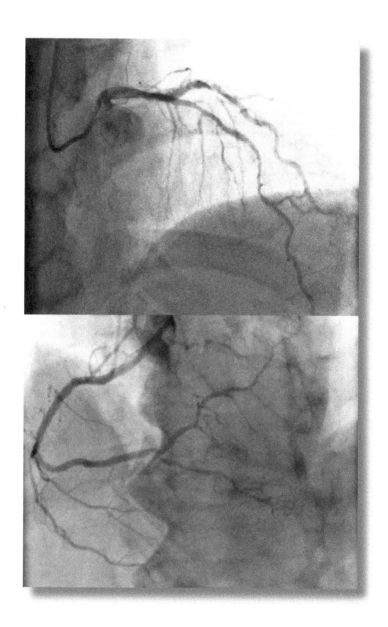

REFERENCES AND CREDITS

Introduction
- Website: www.AWorldWithoutHeartDisease.com
- Website: https://en.wikipedia.org/wiki/Duane_Graveline
- Website: https://spacedoc.com/articles/my-statin-story
- Website: www.SpaceDoc.com
- Website: https://spacedoc.com/sitemap.php
- Website: https://www.thincs.org/
- Website: http://tinyurl.com/y84s66rg, also https://spacedoc.com/articles/statins-and-coq10-deficiency

CHAPTER ONE – The End
- U.S. Patent # 5278189 (https://tinyurl.com/y6udkce8 also https://patents.google.com/patent/US278189) – filed in 1994 by American scientist Linus Pauling and German doctor Matthias Rath, MD, and titled "Prevention and treatment of occlusive cardiovascular disease with ascorbate and substances that inhibit the binding of lipoprotein (A)"

- Reference: "Vitamin C Material: Where to Start, What to Watch"– Commentary by Tom Taylor (https://tinyurl.com/ybrrh8gt also http://orthomolecular.org/resources/omns/v13n20.shtml)

CHAPTER TWO – What Happens If I Stop This Protocol?
- AWorldWithoutHeartDisease.com
- *Why Stomach Acid Is Good for You* (Amazon Kindle, http://tinyurl.com/y73jyudm also https://www.amazon.com/Why-Stomach-Acid-Good-You/dp/0871319314) by *Jonathan V. Wright M.D.*, and *Lane Lenard Ph.D.* http://en.wikipedia.org/wiki/Linus_Pauling - cite_note-0

CHAPTER THREE – Was Linus Pauling Nuts?
- Wikipedia, "Linus Carl Pauling (February 28, 1901 - August 19, 1994)http://en.wikipedia.org/wiki/Linus_Pauling - cite_note-0
(https://en.wikipedia.org/wiki/Linus_Pauling)
- Video of Pauling at age 91: https://tinyurl.com/yb2dpjbm also https://www.youtube.com/watch?v=2bymKIPaTws
- Book: *Vitamin C, the Common Cold, and the Flu* [Paperback] by Linus Pauling (https://tinyurl.com/yafzjcsy also https://www.amazon.com/Vitamin-C-Common-Cold-Flu/dp/0716703610/ref=pd_sim_14_2?_encoding=UTF8&psc=1&refRID=DC8NH3BBVP5BEQAMCGGA)
- Efforts to discredit Pauling can be seen at https://tinyurl.com/ydzykbua also https://www.cancertutor.com/war_pauling/
- Tribute video to Pauling: https://tinyurl.com/nahbrtl also https://www.youtube.com/watch?v=OfuXHJh3LMY

– British researchers on Vitamin C: https://tinyurl.com/ycmfs4e8 also https://www.tandfonline.com/doi/abs/10.1080/13590840802305423

CHAPTER FOUR – What did Pauling and Rath learn about Heart Disease?

– Book, *How to Live Longer and Feel Better* (May 1, 2006) [Hardcover and Paperback] by Linus Pauling (https://tinyurl.com/ya5pejjb also https://www.amazon.com/How-Live-Longer-Feel-Better/dp/0870710966)

– Book: *Vitamin C and the Common Cold*: https://tinyurl.com/ycf3ytwb also https://www.amazon.com/Vitamin-Common-Cold-Linus-Pauling/dp/1568496699

– Website: https://tinyurl.com/ya7pw89c also http://www.orthomolecular.org/index.shtml

– Wikipedia: Quantum chemistry, http://tinyurl.com/yaz2btg9 also https://en.wikipedia.org/wiki/Quantum_chemistry

– Wikipedia: Molecular biology (http://tinyurl.com/lhclspj also https://en.wikipedia.org/wiki/Molecular_biology)

– "Unified Theory" of heart disease (https://tinyurl.com/y9f5wy63 also https://paulingblog.wordpress.com/2017/02/15/the-unified-theory-of-human-cardiovascular-disease/)

– Matthias Rath (https://tinyurl.com/ydcqa6y3 also https://en.wikipedia.org/wiki/Matthias_Rath)

– Rath Foundation critique of Wikipedia article (http://tinyurl.com/ponzgvw also https://www.dr-rath-foundation.org/)

- Wikipedia, "Scurvy" (https://tinyurl.com/mnh7shg also https://en.wikipedia.org/wiki/Scurvy)
- Book, The Vitamin C Connection ((https://tinyurl.com/y9gpph56 also https://www.amazon.com/Vitamin-C-Connection-Cheraskin/dp/0060380241)
- Naturopath and Pauling advocate/chronicler Owen R. Fonorow (https://tinyurl.com/ycdzvpr9 also http://www.internetwks.com/owen/HeartCureRD.htm)
- Online publication, Human Gene Therapy (http://tinyurl.com/nra66an also http://online.liebertpub.com/doi/abs/10.1089/hum.2008.0106)
- Lipoprotein a (Lp(a)): http://tinyurl.com/y8zfpa4f also https://www.ncbi.nlm.nih.gov/pmc/articles/PMC1853362/
- Lp(a) Foundation at https://tinyurl.com/ybw27kla also http://www.lipoproteinafoundation.org/page/StatinsandLpa
- Paper: Lipoprotein (a) in the arterial wall – U. Beisiegel, A. Niendorf, K. Wolf, T. Reblin and M. Rath. European Heart Journal (1990) 11 (Suppl. E), 174-183 (website: http://tinyurl.com/oc9x63j also https://www.dr-rath-foundation.org/)
- Publication: *Circulation* 74, No. 4, 758-765, 1986, Association of levels of lipoprotein Lp(a), plasma lipids, and other lipoproteins with coronary artery disease documented by angiography (https://tinyurl.com/ycmsqc6t also http://circ.ahajournals.org/content/circulationaha/74/4/758.full.pdf)
- New York Times article, "New Heart Studies Question the Value Of Opening Arteries," published March 21,

2004 (http://tinyurl.com/ou74ek6 also http://www.
nytimes.com/2004/03/21/us/new-heart-studies-question-
the-value-of-opening-arteries.html?pagewanted=4)

– Paper, "Comparing the 'Lipid Theory' with the 'Unified
Theory": https://tinyurl.com/yc7k2yzb also http://www.
ourhealthcoop.com/pdf/MikeCiell_unified_theory.pdf

CHAPTER FIVE – Why the "Pauling Protocol" Works

– YouTube Video: "*Vitamin C, Heart Disease, Cancer,
Collagen, Linus Pauling*" (https://tinyurl.com/yb2dpjbm
also https://www.youtube.com/watch?v=2bymKIPaTws)

– HealthCeltral.com report: "Lipoprotein Testing: Why
it's So Important and Where You Can Get it Done (web
link: http://tinyurl.com/q4q2pe8 also https://www.
healthcentral.com/article/lipoprotein-testing-why-its-so-
important-and-where-you-can-get-it-done)

– Quest Diagnostics was recently fined $6 million (https://
tinyurl.com/ya7smfab also https://www.genomeweb.
com/business-news/quest-pay-6-million-settle-kickback-
unnecessary-testing-allegations-berkeley-heartlab) because
the subsidiary it acquired, Berkeley HeartLab, had been
bribing doctors and patients.

– Searches for Berkeley now lead to this web
pages like this: https://tinyurl.com/y849868o
also https://www.phillipsandcohen.com/
quest-diagnostics-whistleblower-settlement-blood-tests/.

– U.S. patent # 5230996, "treatment prior to
transplantation" (https://tinyurl.com/yayupkvz also http://
www.internetwks.com/pauling/lpatent2.html)

- New World Encyclopedia, Vitamin C Chemical Structure https://tinyurl.com/y9mf9rqr also http://www. newworldencyclopedia.org/entry/Vitamin_C
- About.com Chemistry, Chemical Structure of L-Lysine http://tinyurl.com/od35yha also https://www.thoughtco. com/amino-acid-structures-4054180
- PubChem, Chemical Structure of L-Proline https:// tinyurl.com/y8jacxz4 also https://pubchem.ncbi.nlm.nih. gov/compound/L-proline#section=Top

CHAPTER SIX – What Pauling and others have suggested adding to the Protocol

- Pauling's recommended supplementation as of 1986, from the website Cancer Survival (https://tinyurl.com/ y7eeydg6 also http://www.cancersurvival.com/help_ pauling.html)
- Jonathan Campbell website (https://tinyurl.com/y8k4urvf also http://www.healthy-again.net/cvd.htm)
- Thomas E. Levy, MD, JD website (https://tinyurl.com/ y7nzxk7s also https://www.peakenergy.com/index.html)
- Book: Thomas E. Levy, MD, JD, *Stop America's #1 Killer* (https://tinyurl.com/yccprp8q also https://www.medfoxpub.com/medicalnews/ product/S-SAK/Stop-Americas-#1-Killer/ The-path-around-coronary-heart-disease/)

CHAPTER SEVEN – But What About Cholesterol?

- Malcolm Kendrick, MD (MbChB MRCGP), *2007 article,* "Have we been conned about cholesterol?" published in the U.K. Daily Mail On Line (http://tinyurl.com/5bvjf4

also http://www.dailymail.co.uk/health/article-430682/
Have-conned-cholesterol.html)

— Report: "Blood Coagulation Abnormalities Produced
by Feeding Cholesterol to Rabbits" (web link: http://
tinyurl.com/oebchp2 also http://onlinelibrary.wiley.com/
doi/10.1111/j.1365-2141.1957.tb05535.x/abstract)

— Discussion of LDL and HDL: (http://tinyurl.com/bryr5q5
also https://www.livestrong.com/article/401250-how-does-
ldl-hdl-differ-structurally-functionally/)

— Book: *The Great Cholesterol Con,* Malcolm Kendrick M.D.
(https://tinyurl.com/y83xok6a also https://www.amazon.
com/Great-Cholesterol-Really-Causes-Disease-ebook/dp/
B0078XGXQM)

— YouTube video: Dr. Kendrick with his graph comparing
cholesterol levels in specific populations against deaths
from heart disease in those same countries (http://tinyurl.
com/nfe7c7r also https://www.youtube.com/watch?v=i8SS
CNaaDcE&feature=player_embedded)

— Spoof cartoon supporting Dr. Kendrick's work (https://
tinyurl.com/q5n3ony also https://www.youtube.com/
watch?v=GqdzJLOQM2I)

— Dr. Duane Graveline, MD (http://spacedoc.com/)

— Books: *Lipitor, Thief of Memory* (https://tinyurl.com/
y94xp8g9 also https://www.amazon.com/Lipitor-
Thief-Memory-Duane-Graveline/dp/1424301629),
and, *Statin Drugs Side Effects* (https://tinyurl.com/
ydgouev7 also https://www.amazon.com/Statin-Drugs-
Effects-Misguided-Cholesterol/dp/0970081790), Duane
Graveline, M.D., MPH

- "Third Report of the Expert Panel on Detection, Evaluation, and Treatment of High Blood Cholesterol in Adults (Adult Treatment Panel III)." (https://tinyurl.com/yb4ft282 also https://www.nhlbi.nih.gov/files/docs/guidelines/atp3xsum.pdf)

- National Institutes of Health ATP III Update 2004: Financial Disclosure (reveals financial connections of those setting cholesterol target levels with the companies that manufacture and sell cholesterol drugs. (2018 Update NOTE: The NIH has removed links to this data from the Internet. However, you can find that information recreated at https://tinyurl.com/ybhv734 also http://wholehealthsource.blogspot.in/2008/08/conflict-of-interest.html).

- National Institutes of Health, May 26, 2011 (https://tinyurl.com/ycyb9bgb also https://www.nih.gov/news-events/news-releases/nih-stops-clinical-trial-combination-cholesterol-treatment)

- Reuters report, "Low 'good' cholesterol doesn't cause heart attacks," (http://tinyurl.com/y7yrspv8 also https://www.reuters.com/article/us-low-cholesterol/low-good-cholesterol-doesnt-cause-heart-attacks-idUSTRE7B02S820111201)

- November, 2012, Journal of Clinical Endocrinology and Metabolism (http://tinyurl.com/oh5stp9 also https://academic.oup.com/jcem/article/97/2/E248/2836563)

- Dr. Graveline's chronicle of statin-related health issues leading to his death (http://tinyurl.com/y8294xrd also https://spacedoc.com/articles/my-statin-story)

- Dr. Graveline's final book, *The Dark Side of Statins* (https://tinyurl.com/yc5blx9d also https://spacedoc.com/articles/my-statin-story)
- His own synopsis of the book (https://tinyurl.com/yck99nr3 also https://spacedoc.com/articles/the-dark-side-of-statins)

CHAPTER EIGHT – How Come Drugs Seem to "Cure" Only SYMPTOMS?

- Website: "Outlaw the 'Business with Disease': The Chemnitz Program" (http://tinyurl.com/p63k676 also https://www.dr-rath-foundation.org/)
- U.S. Food and Drug Administration website, "Current Drug Shortages" (http://tinyurl.com/ycwg5lva also https://www.accessdata.fda.gov/scripts/drugshortages/default.cfm)
- Subscribe to the FDA site (https://tinyurl.com/yapgqos6 also http://go.fda.gov/subscriptionmanagement)
- Institute for Safe Medication Practices paper on shortages of prescription drugs (https://tinyurl.com/y7kptoq4 also https://www.ismp.org/newsletters/acutecare/articles/20100923.asp)
- Public Citizen report on pharmaceutical industry profit (http://tinyurl.com/yd8yv6u6 also https://www.citizen.org/sites/default/files/pharma-profits-and-r-and-d-report.pdf).
- Wall Street Journal (http://tinyurl.com/q9o5kag also https://www.wsj.com/articles/partnership-takes-aim-at-curing-hiv-aids-1431309601) in May 2015, Glaxo announced it was funding a joint venture to "cure" AIDS

- Website, "What You Need to Know About the Fraudulent Nature of the Pharmaceutical Investment Business With Disease (http://tinyurl.com/o7heeqw also https://www.dr-rath-foundation.org/)
- Website, "Case Study of Scientific Corruption" (http://tinyurl.com/yd86jdy3 also https://www.cancertutor.com/war_pauling/)
- Website, "War Between Orthodox And Alternative Medicine" (https://tinyurl.com/ycyl2prf also https://www.cancertutor.com/warbetween/)
- Orlando Sentinel article, "Florida doctors taking millions of dollars in Big Pharma money," (http://tinyurl.com/pspzavw also http://articles.orlandosentinel.com/2011-09-07/health/os-doctors-pharma-list-20110907_1_drug-companies-research-companies-florida-doctors)
- Centers for Medicare & Medicaid Services (CMS), "Find your Doctor's Payments" (https://tinyurl.com/nypkyze also https://openpaymentsdata.cms.gov/)
- ProPublica website, "Dollars for Docs" (https://tinyurl.com/khe9n8y also https://projects.propublica.org/docdollars/)
- Bradenton, FL, Times on Sunday, Nov 01, 2015, "How Big Pharma Gets to Have Its Cake and Eat it Too (http://tinyurl.com/y9bd5z9u also http://thebradentontimes.com/how-big-pharma-gets-to-have-its-cake-and-eat-it-too-p14038-137.htm?utm_source=Readers&utm_campaign=0a7f02d1f0-RSS_EMAIL_CAMPAIGN&utm_medium=email&utm_term=0_1d2bd00576-0a7f02d1f0-25447825)

- "Pharmaceutical companies argue that they need to gouge in the U.S." (http://tinyurl. com/y7nqmzhe also https://www.reuters.com/ article/us-health-pharmaceuticals-cancer-usa/ exclusive-americans-overpaying-hugely-for-cancer-drugs-study-idUSKCN0RM1EC20150922)
- "Big Pharma sprinkled more than $50 million on candidates in the 2012 presidential election cycle (http:// tinyurl.com/nnz2ccf also http://www.truth-out.org/news/ item/33010-how-much-of-big-pharma-s-massive-profits-are-used-to-influence-politicians)
- 2017 update: http://tinyurl.com/y9nmahrj also https:// www.opensecrets.org/lobby/indusclient.php?id=h04)
- Hundreds of millions handed out to doctors for "speaking fees" (http://tinyurl.com/ycexseut also https://www. nytimes.com/2014/10/01/business/Database-of-payments-to-doctors-by-drug-and-medical-device-makers.html?_r=1)
- 9 out of the 10 top pharmaceutical companies spend more money on sales and marketing than R&D (http:// tinyurl.com/gpkovzy also http://naturalsociety.com/ research-development-new-drugs-not-paying-off-6321/)
- Eye-popping compensation for CEOs (http://tinyurl. com/zoxqav2 also https://www.fiercepharma.com/ special-report/top-20-highest-paid-biopharma-ceos)

CHAPTER NINE – Why What You Don't Know About Statin Drugs Could, a) Cripple You, or b) Wreck Your Brain or c) Kill You

- Website of Duane Graveline, MD, MPH, on the Netherlands study (http://tinyurl.com/ya9serjk also https:// spacedoc.com/articles/the-netherlands-radar-survey)

- Lipitor Official Website (http://www.lipitor.com/)
- New York Times (http://tinyurl.com/ofxy5za also https://
  well.blogs.nytimes.com/2014/05/05/a-new-womens-issue-
  statins/?_r=0) [13th paragraph)]
- Rhabdomyolysis explained by PubMed Health (https://
  tinyurl.com/y7mnwbeq also https://www.ncbi.nlm.nih.
  gov/pubmedhealth/PMHT0024696/)
- YouTube video, "An Update on Demonization and
  Deception in Research on Saturated Fat," (http://
  tinyurl.com/gkv7cju also https://www.youtube.com/
  watch?v=yX1vBA9bLNk) by Professor David M. Diamond
- Dr. Graveline's book, *Statin Drugs Side Effects,* referenced
  previously
- "Statin Damage to the Mevalonate Pathway,"
  Dr. Graveline (https://tinyurl.com/
  yb376dwv also https://spacedoc.com/articles/
  statins-and-the-mevalonate-pathway)
- FDA notice that statin drugs are related to memory loss
  (http://tinyurl.com/yaybv2x8 also https://www.fda.gov/
  drugs/drugsafety/ucm293101.htm)
- AARP article, "10 Drugs That May Cause Memory Loss"
  (http://tinyurl.com/m6mdmah also https://www.aarp.org/
  health/brain-health/info-05-2013/drugs-that-may-cause-
  memory-loss.html#quest1)
- Big Pharma is after your kids: (http://tinyurl.com/2f9kg7d
  also https://articles.mercola.com/sites/articles/
  archive/2010/07/20/the-truth-about-statin-drugs-revealed.
  aspx). See section, "Parents Beware: Outrageous Push to
  Put Kids on Statin Drugs!"
- "A Recipe for Alzheimer's Disease" (http://

tinyurl.com/yc7x84jd also https://spacedoc.com/
articles/a-recipe-for-alzheimers)

— Dr. Mercola's interview (http://tinyurl.com/ykckdww
also https://articles.mercola.com/sites/articles/
archive/2009/12/05/Does-High-Cholesterol-REALLY-
Cause-Heart-Disease.aspx) with the founder of THINCS,
The International Network of Cholesterol Skeptics

— Website for The International Network of Cholesterol
Skeptics (THINCS) (http://www.thincs.org/news.htm)

**Following is a suggested reading list taken from the website for
The International Network of Cholesterol Skeptics**

— John von Radowitz, (The Independent): 85% of new drugs
'offer few benefits' (http://tinyurl.com/2c8atl8 also http://
www.independent.co.uk/life-style/health-and-families/
health-news/85-of-new-drugs-offer-few-benefits-2054972.
html)

— Christopher Hudson (Telegraph), Wonder drug that stole
my memory (http://tinyurl.com/ybwsdomt also https://
www.telegraph.co.uk/news/health/4974840/Wonder-drug-
that-stole-my-memory.html). Statins have been hailed as
a miracle cure for cholesterol, but little is known about
their side effects. Read also the comments that follow the
article, but beware, they are scary.

— Melinda Wenner Moyer (Scientific American),
It's Not Dementia, It's Your Heart Medication:
Cholesterol Drugs and Memory. Why cholesterol
drugs might affect memory. (http://tinyurl.com/
zjh2gsj also https://www.scientificamerican.com/article/
its-not-dementia-its-your-heart-medication/)

- Tom Naughton, Big Fat Fiasco: how the misguided fear of saturated fat created a nation of obese diabetics (http://tinyurl.com/22q7z86 also http://www.fathead-movie.com/index.php/2010/10/28/video-of-the-big-fat-fiasco-speech/). A humourous speech with a serious content. Five parts, on Youtube
- Uffe Ravnskov, Ignore the Awkward! How the Cholesterol Myths are Kept Alive (http://tinyurl.com/y9ntzskw also https://www.amazon.com/Ignore-Awkward-Cholesterol-Myths-Alive/dp/1453759409/ref=sr_1_1?ie=UTF8&s=books&qid=1288080387&sr=1-1). A book.about how prominent scientists have turned white into black by ignoring all conflicting observations; by twisting and exaggerating trivial findings; by citing studies with opposing results in a way to make them look supportive; and by ignoring or scorning the work of critical scientists. Includes a short and simplified version of his previous book
- Denise Minger, The China Study: Fact or Fallacy (http://tinyurl.com/y8p77w3d also https://deniseminger.com/2010/07/07/the-china-study-fact-or-fallac/). Is the book by that title, authored by Colin Campbell, really "one of the most important books about nutrition ever written", as stated on the cover by Dean Ornish? Or is it, rather, one of the most misleading? Read Minger's review.
- David H. Freeman, Lies, Damned Lies and Medical Science (http://tinyurl.com/mrqpvgs also https://www.theatlantic.com/magazine/archive/2010/11/lies-damned-lies-and-medical-science/308269/). The Atlantic Nov. 2010

- PublicCitizen, Dec 16, 2010: Rapidly Increasing Criminal and Civil Monetary Penalties Against the Pharmaceutical Industry: 1991 to 2010 (http://tinyurl.com/ycbjkgpo also https://www.citizen.org/our-work/health-and-safety/rapidly-increasing-criminal-and-civil-monetary-penalties-against)
- Malcolm Kendrick, The Cholesterol Myth exposed (http://tinyurl.com/y84uvf9u also https://www.youtube.com/watch?v=i8SSCNaaDcE). A short YouTube presentation
- *Lipitor Paradox*, A funny but also sad YouTube movie (http://tinyurl.com/q5n3ony also https://www.youtube.com/watch?v=GqdzJLOQM2I) in support of Kendrick's findings.
- Emily Deans, Low Cholesterol and Suicide (http://tinyurl.com/yam8z9fd also https://www.psychologytoday.com/blog/evolutionary-psychiatry/201103/low-cholesterol-and-suicide).
- Dwight D Lundell, The Statin Scam (http://tinyurl.com/y9j4zf8m also https://spacedoc.com/articles/statin-scam). A view from an experienced thoracic surgeon.
- Stephanie Seneff, How Statins Really Work Explains Why They Don't Really Work (http://tinyurl.com/6zdjp9d also http://people.csail.mit.edu/seneff/why_statins_dont_really_work.html).

CHAPTER TEN – Women and Statin Drugs

- Book: *The Great Cholesterol Con* by Malcolm Kendrick; John Blake Publishing (https://tinyurl.com/y8zsssnq also https://drmalcolmkendrick.org/books-by-dr-malcolm-kendrick/the-great-cholesterol-con/)

- *Time Magazine* article, "Do Statins Work Equally for Men and Women? (web link: http://tinyurl.com/nn5bu94 also http://content.time.com/time/magazine/article/0,9171,1973295,00.html#ixzz1YKfbXl2Y)

- *Consumer Reports Magazine* article, "Women and statins: When the drugs may not make sense" (http://tinyurl.com/nkcrw7g also https://www.consumerreports.org/cro/2010/06/women-and-statins-when-the-drugs-may-not-make-sense/index.htm)

- Website: "Statins risk for women: Taking cholesterol-lowering drug for more than ten years 'doubles chances of the most common breast cancer'" (http://tinyurl.com/ljc8866 also http://www.dailymail.co.uk/health/article-2370825/Statins-risk-women-Taking-cholesterol-lowering-drug-years-doubles-chances-common-breast-cancer.html)

- Statins for Women? Not for My Patients (http://tinyurl.com/muqo3ju also https://www.huffingtonpost.com/kelly-brogan-md/women-statins_b_4283650.html)

- The New York Times blog, May 5, 2014 (http://tinyurl.com/ofxy5za also https://well.blogs.nytimes.com/2014/05/05/a-new-womens-issue-statins/?_r=0)

- Dr. Mark Hyman, MD, October 18, 2014 (http://tinyurl.com/mh2dxu4 also http://drhyman.com/blog/2012/01/19/why-women-should-stop-their-cholesterol-lowering-medication/)

- Catharine Paddock PhD, Medical News Today, March 16, 2017 (https://tinyurl.com/y8g7dnaq also https://www.medicalnewstoday.com/articles/316409.php)

- Joe Graedon, The People's Pharmacy online (https://tinyurl.com/yc2wg2jg also https://www.peoplespharmacy.com/2018/01/25/should-everyone-over-65-take-a-statin-to-prevent-a-heart-attack/)

CHAPTER ELEVEN – If Your Doctor Says "Don't Try This," Find Another Doctor

- "Vitamin C And The Law, A Personal Viewpoint" by Thomas E. Levy, M.D., J.D. (http://www.whale.to/a/vitc45.html) "This article may be reprinted free of charge provided 1) that there is clear attribution to the Orthomolecular Medicine News Service, and 2) that both the OMNS free subscription link at http://www.orthomolecular.org/forms/omns_subscribe.shtml http://www.cihfimediaservices.org/12all/lt/t_go.php?i=118&e=MjUwNjU=&l=-http–orthomolecular.org/subscribe.htmland also the OMNS archive link at http://orthomolecular.org/library/jom/index.shtml are included.
- "Vitamin C and Sepsis, The genie is now out of the bottle" (https://tinyurl.com/ycoa8j3r also http://orthomolecular.org/resources/omns/v13n12.shtml)

APPENDIX A – My Actual Daily Intake, And Why I Take All Those Pills

- Orthomolecular.org News Service:
- "No Deaths from Vitamins. None." (https://tinyurl.com/y7gap6ng also http://orthomolecular.org/resources/omns/v13n01.shtml)

- "No Deaths from Supplements. No Deaths from Minerals or Amino Acids. No Deaths from Homeopathics or Herbs." (https://tinyurl.com/ycg6j3ql also http://orthomolecular.org/resources/omns/v13n02.shtml).
- Website, Orthomolecular.org, "This article may be reprinted free of charge provided 1) that there is clear attribution to the Orthomolecular Medicine News Service, and 2) that both the OMNS free subscription link at http://www.orthomolecular.org/forms/omns_subscribe.shtml http://www.cihfimediaservices.org/12all/lt/t_go.php?i=118&e=MjUwNjU=&l=-http–orthomolecular.org/subscribe.htmland also the OMNS archive link at http://orthomolecular.org/library/jom/index.shtml are included.
- Website, Medical Knowledge Base ("MedKB"), "Drug Errors Send 700,000 to ER Every Year" (http://tinyurl.com/o4bts72 also http://www.foxnews.com/story/2006/10/18/drug-errors-send-700000-to-er-every-year.html)
- Consumer Labs discussion on synthetic fish oil (https://tinyurl.com/y9b6m83c also https://www.consumerlab.com/answers/are-fish-oil-supplements-as-good-as-prescription-fish-oil-like-lovaza/Lovaza_cost/)
- Learn about Consumer Labs and membership (http://tinyurl.com/r2gjy also https://www.consumerlab.com/aboutcl.asp)
- Mayo Clinic discussion on vitamin E: https://tinyurl.com/y97cnhw3 also https://www.mayoclinic.org/drugs-supplements-vitamin-e/art-20364144
- Booklet, Prostate Disorders and Natural Medicine, By Rita Elkins (web link: http://tinyurl.com/q2o5dnc,

also https://books.google.co.in/books?id=hPSE6g51
HRIC&pg=PA20&lpg=PA20&dq=Prostate+gland,+
Bee+Pollen+and+Zinc&source=bl&ots=nDMZNcuK
5J&sig=Jr_KrhPAlzbrejFZjtG-cT_pPOI&hl=en&ei=
xKmRToTdMpK2tgfFwtmQDA&sa=X&oi=book_
result&ct=result&redir_esc=y#v=onepage&q=Prostate
gland%2C Bee Pollen and Zinc&f=false)

APPENDIX B – Will You Let The U.S. Government Take Away Your Vitamins And Supplements?

— Orthomolecular Medicine News Service, January 5, 2017 (https://tinyurl.com/ycg6j3ql also http://orthomolecular. org/resources/omns/v13n02.shtml)

— Centers for Disease Control and Prevention on Adverse Drug Event Monitoring (http://tinyurl.com/pwwhgvo also https://www.cdc.gov/MedicationSafety/program_focus_ activities.html)

— New York Times (http://tinyurl.com/4os6qmz also http:// www.nytimes.com/2011/01/11/science/11aging.html)

— "Dietary Supplement Labeling Act of 2011" (S. 1310) (https://tinyurl.com/yctn7bzj also https://www.congress. gov/bill/112th-congress/senate-bill/1310), and reintroduced in 2013 (https://tinyurl.com/ya92kdcl also https://www. govtrack.us/congress/bills/113/s1425/text)

— FDA "Dietary Supplements Guidance Documents & Regulatory Information" (https://tinyurl.com/y9q4v2a5 also https://www.fda.gov/Food/GuidanceRegulation/ GuidanceDocumentsRegulatoryInformation/ DietarySupplements/default.htm)

- Writer and Critical Care Nurse Byron J. Richards articles regarding Durbin and the FDA http://tinyurl.com/p7q7cl7 also http://www.newswithviews.com/Richards/byron213.htm http://tinyurl.com/3z4q9cd also http://www.newswithviews.com/Richards/byron211.htm http://tinyurl.com/3zmawek also http://www.newswithviews.com/Richards/byron210.htm
- Book, 2015 attacks on dietary supplements https://tinyurl.com/ybukmx6e also http://www.anh-usa.org/new-study-totally-misrepresents-adverse-events-related-to-dietary-supplements/

"About the graph on the Back Cover"
- The WHO MONICA project is described here: https://tinyurl.com/y9hvjtth also http://www.epi.umn.edu/cvdepi/essay/the-monica-project/

Websites Studied in Researching this Book
(Not in any particular order)
- The Cure for Heart Disease: Condensed by Owen R. Fonorow, Copyright 2004 http://www.internetwks.com/owen/HeartCureRD.htm
- http://paulingtherapy.com/
- http://www.internetwks.com/pauling/index.html
- http://www.practicingmedicinewithoutalicense.com/protocol/
- Pauling video on the body's ability to absorb vitamin C: http://www.youtube.com/watch?v=QXiUcU3rz3s

Pauling on his research with Rath:

- https://www.youtube.com/watch?v=2bymKIPaTws
- "Lipoprotein (a) in the arterial wall," U. Beisiegel, A. Niendorf, K. Wolf, T. Reblin and M. Rath *EUROPEAN HEART JOURNAL (1990) 11 (SUPPL. E), 174-183* http://www4.dr-rath-foundation.org/THE_FOUNDATION/About_Dr_Matthias_Rath/publications/pub03.htm

Previously listed on http://store.ourhealthcoop.com/Heart_Plus_p/he.htm:

Studies:

1. The Linus Pauling Institute: Micronutrient Information Center. http://lpi.oregonstate.edu/infocenter/vitamins/vitaminC/index.html

2. Rath M and Pauling L. (1994) U.S. Patent # 5278189; Prevention and treatment of occlusive cardiovascular disease with ascorbate and substances that inhibit the binding of lipoprotein (A) https://patents.google.com/patent/US5278189

3. Rath, M and Pauling, L. (1992) "A unified theory of human cardiovascular disease leading the way to the abolition of this disease as a cause for human mortality. http://momgil.cafe24.com/wp-content/uploads/2010/03/UnifiedTheory1.pdf?ckattempt=1

4. Rath M and Pauling L. (1991) Solution to the puzzle of human cardiovascular disease: Its primary cause is ascorbate deficiency, leading to the deposition of lipoprotein (a) and fibrinogen/fibrin in the vascular wall. http://tinyurl.com/yek5wjb also https://www.dr-rath-foundation.org/

5. Rath M and Pauling L. (1990) "Hypothesis: lipoprotein(a) is a surrogate for ascorbate." Proc Natl

Acad Sci U S A. 1990 Aug;87(16):6204-7. Erratum in: Proc Natl Acad Sci U S A 1991 Dec 15;88(24):11588. http://tinyurl.com/pjrk7qd also https://www.ncbi.nlm.nih.gov/pmc/articles/PMC54501/?tool=pubmed

6. Rath M and Pauling L. (1990) "Immunological evidence for the accumulation of lipoprotein(a) in the atherosclerotic lesion of the hypoascorbemic guinea pig." Proc Natl Acad Sci U S A. 1990 Dec;87(23):9388-90. http://tinyurl.com/ob2yqw9 also https://www.ncbi.nlm.nih.gov/pmc/articles/PMC55170/?tool=pubmed

− Orthomolecular News Service 9OMNS)

− http://www.orthomolecular.org/resources/omns/index.shtml

− Vitamin C and The Law. A Personal Viewpoint by Thomas E. Levy, M.D., J.D. http://www.whale.to/a/vitc45.html

− Dr. Levy's Website http://www.tomlevymd.com/

− Vitamin C Foundation's Videos of Pauling and others. http://www.vitamincfoundation.org/videos/

− Vitamin C Saves Dying Man http://healthimpactnews.com/2013/vitamin-c-saves-man-dying-of-viral-pneumonia/

− IF YOU HAVE RECENTLY HEARD THAT VITAMINS ARE HARMFUL, you may want to read this: http://www.doctoryourself.com/safety.html

− Addendum A: E-Scripts Drug Digest: https://www.express-scripts.com/medco/consumer/ehealth/druginfo/dlmain.jsp?WC=N

− Coming full circle, there is my own website: http://aworldwithoutheartdisease.com/

ABOUT THE GRAPH ON THE BACK COVER

Americans typically describe cholesterol levels in milligrams per deciliter, commonly expressed as mg/dl. In other parts of the world and among scientists, the measure often used is millimoles per litre (*mmol*/L). The factor to calculate between the two is 38.7. So, the figures in red on the graph translate as follows:

6.5 *mmol*/L = 252 mg/dl (supposedly dangerous levels)

5.5 *mmol*/L = 213 mg/dl (supposedly borderline)

4.5 *mmol*/L = 174 mg/dl (supposedly "least likely" to incur heart attacks)

Death rates (the black numbers and line) are per 100,000 population.

Study those World Health Organization (WHO) numbers, and draw your own conclusions. The WHO MONICA project is described here: https://tinyurl.com/y9hvjtth

PHOTOS ON NEXT PAGE

Photos on opposite page are X-rays of my heart's arteries, taken during an exploratory angiogram conducted at Florida Hospital Orlando on July 27, 2011. I turned 70 years old in January 2012. A nurse in the "cath lab" said she hoped her own arteries right then looked as clean as mine. The cardiologist who performed the procedure (not my normal heart doctor) proclaimed my heart healthy (*"free of obstructive disease,"* were his written words) as did my family doctor, based on the cardiologist's report.

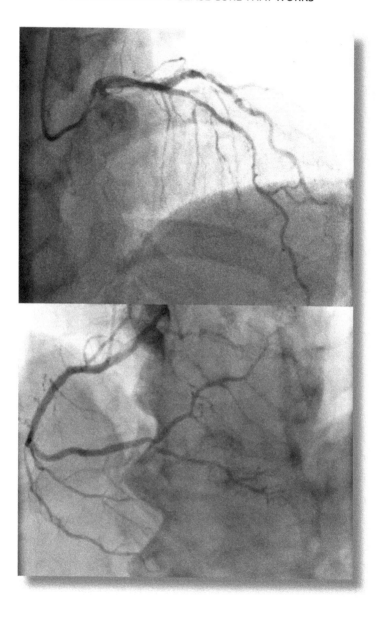

The upper photo is of my Left Anterior Descending (LAD) artery bundle, commonly known to heart doctors as "the widow maker." At one point, it contained a blockage of 85 percent. Later, my heart became home to three metal mesh stents. The only damage this cardiologist could now find involved those stents.

The lower photo displays the clean arteries on the back side of my heart. That straight line is actually the X-ray image of the catheter that was inserted through my thigh, into my femoral artery and then threaded into my heart. Through it, contrasting dye was injected that would then light up the X-rays. Dark spots are intersections, where a branch attaches to the main vessel. They are dark because we are looking into the trunk of a wide open vessel, so the camera picks up a greater amount of dye in the blood passing through that point.

My change in heart health occurred *after* 17 years of bad reactions to every statin drug (Lipitor was the last, and the worst). It was only after I had run out of statin options that I turned in desperation to searching the Internet. That's how I discovered the 1994 patent that changed my life. It might change yours. That's what this book is about.

For more details, and to view pages from my actual medical records, visit my website, www.AWorldWithoutHeartDisease.com.

Lightning Source UK Ltd.
Milton Keynes UK
UKHW020928271220
375968UK00010B/517